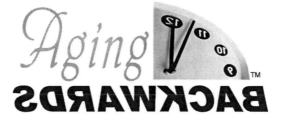

Aging Backwards: Secrets to Staying Young

Jackie Silver

Please read: The entire contents of this book are based upon the opinions of Jackie Silver, unless otherwise noted, and for educational purposes only. The information and products mentioned in this book are not intended to diagnose, treat, cure or prevent disease, are not intended as medical advice, and not intended to replace a one-on-one relationship with a qualified healthcare professional, such as a doctor, for when you need one. Be sure to check with your doctor before engaging in any dietary or fitness changes or routines.

ISBN 978-0-9819009-0-2
Cover design and layout by Xavier Rivera
Aging Backwards logo design by Brenda Cutler Boone
Cover photo by Billy "The Kid" Studios
Edited by Pamela Huff
www.agingbackwards.com

Contents

Chapter 4

Chapter 5

Chapter 6

Chapter 7

Chapter 8

Chapter 9

Chapter 10

Chapter 11

Chapter 12

Chapter 13

Chapter 14

Introduction

Getting older may be beyond our control, but how we age is not. I'm Aging Backwards and I invite you to join me. I've written this book to share with you my secrets, tips and shortcuts for looking and feeling younger and it doesn't take superhuman willpower. All it takes are small steps that add up to big results. Some of the tips may surprise you, and some you may have heard before but perhaps you've forgotten them. Don't worry — I'm here to remind you. There's no "magic formula" for Aging Backwards, but if you start with baby steps, before you know it you'll be making strides.

I've always been a voracious reader with a special passion for science and anti-aging. I've interviewed some of the industry's most respected experts on the subject of anti-aging and I share their insights with you throughout this book.

You'll also find plenty of my own observations from real-life experience through trial and error, and maybe through a little blood, sweat and tears. I like to think of myself as the "anti-aging petri dish." I try just about every product, service and new procedure, and then report my results on syndicated television, on radio, in the newspaper and on my Web site. Now I've put it all in one place for you — right here.

I've assembled my best secrets, tips and short-cuts compiled from more than two years of searching and studying and many more years of experimenting with products, services and procedures.

Aging Backwards is about incorporating subtle changes into your life that are within almost anyone's capacity to make. It's about working with what you've got and making a commitment to improving yourself a little bit every single day. But if you do miss a day or you feel like eating that big slice of cake "just this once," so what? Aging Backwards is not about beating yourself up. It's about focusing on the good things you do and doing more of them, more often. Lots of little accomplishments add up to big results and the re-wards are great. The way I've arranged this book, you can flip open to any page and find something that's easy to incorporate into your daily life. Open it up any-where and read for five minutes or 15 minutes. Find a quick tip or take your time. Do whatever motivates you to make positive changes in your life.

Take what you find useful and what speaks to you and forget about the rest. If you look closely enough, you'll find something of interest and value in here that feels right for you.

If you're ready to halt and possibly even reverse the aging process, then read on. I must warn you, though, that Aging Backwards may be habit-forming. You may soon find yourself looking forward to that workout you used to loathe or calling your local med spa to make an appointment.

Life should be an adventure, and adventures are

always best when you approach them with an open, optimistic mind.

As I like to say, it's never too late — or even too early — to start thinking about Aging Backwards. It's tempting to use certain "crutches" to rationalize all the reasons why we can't do this or that. I'm here to help you change your old way of thinking and replace it with new, encouraging, motivating, positive thoughts!

I'm not a doctor, so I'm not giving you any medical advice. But I will tell you what I know, what I've tried and what I've found that works and doesn't work. So, read on and let's turn back the clock — together!

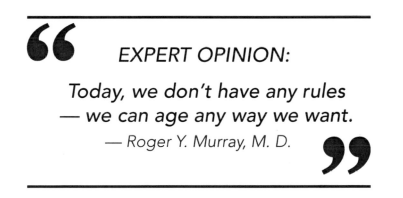

" EXPERT OPINION:

Today, we don't have any rules — we can age any way we want.

— Roger Y. Murray, M. D.

Chapter 1
My Story: Defying Genetics

ne trap many people fall into, thanks to magazines, movies and television, is comparing themselves to others. We engage in all kinds of negative self-talk such as, "These jeans make my butt look big," or "I'll never be as skinny as her." I finally realized none of that matters. What matters to me is that I look and feel the best I can. I started raising my own bar, not to anyone else's standard, but to my own. I decided to eat a healthier diet, add more veggies into my daily meals, exercise more, skip rope and skip the excuses! I'm not a movie star, so I don't compare myself to them.

It wasn't easy getting to this point. I started out in life as an obese child when childhood obesity was virtually unheard of. With the bullies at school picking on the "fat girl," and my own insecurities, I spent the first half of my life battling my demons.

I still have my limitations — we all do — but I'm not letting my genetics stop me from living the best life I can. My father had high blood pressure, high cholesterol and smoked two packs of cigarettes a day. He was overweight and I can't remember ever seeing him exercise in my entire life. My father — a cardiologist — died of a heart attack at 49 years old. I'm 50, but I'm not worrying about a heart attack. I focus on doing the things that help ensure I won't have one. I respect my genetics, but I refuse to allow them to control my life. I enjoy helping others defy their genetics, too. That's why I also speak voluntarily on behalf of the American Heart Association, alerting women to the dangers of heart disease.

Diets and More Diets

Over the years I've tried just about every diet out there. I'm sort of the poster child for dieting. In fact, in the 1990s, I even ended up on posters as the model for Dr. Atkins' low-carb diet.

Eons earlier, as a 13-year-old, I became a lifetime member of Weight Watchers. I've tried the Grapefruit diet, the South Beach diet, Jenny Craig, Slim-Fast, NutriSystem, the Soup diet, L.A. Weight Loss, the Beverly Hills diet, the Zone diet, Atkins ... need I go on? I've even developed a few ridiculous diets of my own. As a teenager, I convinced myself that vanilla yogurt was the perfect diet food and I spent eight months eating nothing else. Another silly idea was my "ice cream diet." That's the one where I ate nothing but ice cream twice a day for a couple of weeks until I almost ended up in a sugar coma. I definitely don't recommend a one-food diet to anyone.

I spent the first 25 years of my life on a roller coaster. I'd be fat and then I'd be skinny; my weight was always on the way up or down. Finally, I learned how to stay thin through healthy lifestyle choices in nutrition and exercise. No matter where you are on the weight scale, I can relate. I was preordained to be fat. I think I was even born fat.

Growing up, we weren't given much in the way of nutritional guidance. Nutrition wasn't really an "in" subject back in the 1960s and '70s. My parents were overweight and our house was full of junk food. I first realized that I was fat at age 7. My mother said one of the other moms at my dance recital pointed me out as "the fat one." How humiliating! A few years later, when I was 10, my mother dragged me to Weight Watchers with her. She was determined we would lose weight together. Naturally, I wanted to continue eating to my heart's content, but instead I had to eat foods I found disgusting, such as liver.

But I did lose weight. In fact, I lost 25 pounds, going from 95 pounds down to 70, which for a 10-year-old is a lot. And I was duly rewarded with a new wardrobe of my favorite "Miss Dorissa" dresses. After a while we quit attending the meetings and I went right back to my old ways. Inevitably, the weight started creeping back.

By the time I was 12 years old, I gained back all the weight I'd lost, plus a lot more. My mother also regained her lost weight, so back to Weight Watchers we went. I remembered how great it felt to be thin and I had matured a little, so I was more interested in it this time around. I didn't follow the program very strictly, but I did manage to lose a few pounds over a couple of months. Then one of the speakers gave a talk that changed my whole attitude. She said, "While we know that everyone cheats, you just need to control your cheating." I happen to be very competitive, so I decided that I "could so" do the program without cheating at all; and that's just what I did.

Over the next nine months, I managed to reach my goal weight. I went from 119 pounds to 83 pounds. I kept the weight off for at least six months and qualified for a lifetime membership with Weight Watchers. Not long after I qualified for lifetime, my mom and I stopped attending the meetings and I fell back into my old eating habits.

By the time I was 15, I had gone from 83 pounds to 150 pounds. No one likes being overweight, and being an overweight teenager in a school full of "prom queens" was not my idea of fun. One day at school I overheard one of the cute, popular boys whisper to his friend, "Jackie would be the prettiest girl at school if she would lose weight." Talk about an eye-opener. That day I decided to go back on a diet and stick to it. But which diet to do this time? I was pretty burned out on Weight Watchers by now.

This brings us to my infamous vanilla yogurt diet. It wasn't a conscious decision on my part to go on a yogurt diet; it sort of evolved because I loved vanilla yogurt. I would eat one, 8-ounce yogurt a day at lunch and make it last half an hour. At home I pretended to eat so my parents wouldn't notice. Eight months later I was down to 110 pounds, and guess what? That adorable boy did ask me out.

That summer, we went on a family vacation to the beach. When my mother saw me in a bikini, she realized I was getting pretty thin. In an effort to tempt me to eat more, she bought me a bag of prunes, which I loved then and still do. After nothing but eight months of yogurt, they tasted delicious. I ate the whole bag and had the runs for the next two days. I didn't eat much during the rest of the vacation, but slowly I started tasting different foods and even though I was forced to expand my diet beyond yogurt, I kept the weight off until my freshman year of college.

Tap Dancing Through Life

Even with all the yo-yo dieting, I was always very active and thoroughly enjoyed tap dancing, riding my bike, jumping rope, climbing trees, gymnastics and tennis. I took tennis lessons for a few years in my teens and actually became quite good at it, but eventually had to quit because the courts were not within walking distance or even biking distance, and I couldn't get consistent rides to my lessons. I'm the middle one of five kids — did I mention that? It was quite a chaotic household with everyone trying to get to their respective classes and lessons.

I also took gymnastics at a professional gym where some Olympic hopefuls trained. When I turned 16 and got my driver's license, the first place I drove to was my gymnastics class in an old airport hangar in Opa-Locka, FL, 17 miles from home each way in a driving rainstorm. I was petrified, but I was determined not to miss my Saturday morning gymnastics lesson. In reality, I was never very good at gymnastics, but I loved it anyway.

Around the time I graduated high school, I joined a gym called Vic Tanny, which had all kinds of shiny workout contraptions I had never seen before, as well as aerobics and stretching classes that sounded very enticing. I was going off to college in New Orleans and the salesperson assured me there was a Vic

Tanny location right near my school. This was right after my vanilla yogurt diet, so I was looking good and wanted to stay that way.

When I arrived in New Orleans for freshman year, one of my first phone calls was to Vic Tanny's, only to find out the branch had closed months before. The closest location was now somewhere in Alabama, so there went my gym membership. Even worse, the company insisted I keep paying for the membership, which I adamantly refused, ruining my credit rating at the tender age of 18. Welcome to adulthood.

Like most freshmen, I wasn't immune to the "freshman 15," only in my case it was more like the "freshman 35." New Orleans was the capital of delectable eating, full of beignets, gumbo, jambalaya and Popeye's Fried Chicken. What was I thinking? I should have gone to UCLA where they were eating sprouts and avocados. Time to shed a few pounds again. This time I replaced yogurt with ice cream. My logic went like this: Since ice cream is basically a liquid, I could lose weight by being on a liquid diet.

I got the idea while walking to my classes because I would pass a little ice cream shop twice a day. How convenient was that? After a couple of weeks of eating only ice cream, I grew so weak that I almost passed out. My roommate found me lying around, too lethargic to even attend classes, and took me to the infirmary. I decided that was a good time to start being a little smarter about nutrition. By that time, I actually had a lot of knowledge about weight loss, not to mention experience — I had already lost a total of 101 pounds by the time I was 17 years old!

Since I couldn't attend the Vic Tanny gym unless I wanted to drive four hours in each direction, I joined my roommate, Sandra, in giving up the dorm elevator for Lent. We were only on the third floor, but you'd be surprised how much exercise you can get without the elevator. We went up and down those stairs at least 10 times a day. Good thing, too, or my freshman 35 would have been more like 55!

I only spent one year in New Orleans, then transferred to University of Florida in Gainesville. This began several years of sloth in the workout department. I landed a job at the local radio station as an on-air personality, which didn't leave me much time to exercise. Even if I could have made time, I basically lost interest because I was so involved with the radio station. Plus, I was still carrying around the extra 35 pounds I had put on in New Orleans, which dampened my enthusiasm for exercise. I kept my extra padding for a few more years, through a few more radio stations and finally, at age 25, I got control of my weight. I went on NutriSystem back when it was considered a "medical diet," and lost 35 pounds. This time, I kept it off. Well, almost.

The only time I ever gained weight again was during my pregnancy, and that was only 30 pounds. Amazingly, after my son was born, the so-called "baby weight" didn't fall off. In fact, when my son was eight months old, I went on Jenny Craig and lost those last 20 pounds. This time, I did keep it off. My son is now 18 and I'm still at my ideal weight.

The Quest for the Holy Scale

Perhaps the most profound change I made over the years was to sever my love affair with the scale. Not completely, mind you, but I became less obsessed with numbers and more focused on the way I felt in my clothes. This became an important theme in my life, and to this day I rarely weigh myself. In fact, I refuse to get on the scale when I go for my yearly well-woman checkup. I know when I need to lose a few pounds and it's usually after the holidays.

That's why every year I do my "Spring Shape-Up," to lose those two or three pounds I gained during the holidays and winter months. I'm like a cavewoman — I put on my winter padding and take it off every spring — but I'm happy to have left the yo-yo dieting behind. Now, I have a love affair with fresh, nutritionally sound food in proper portions. It's one love affair that I intend to continue for a lifetime.

Chapter 2

Aging Backwards Fast Stats

 EXPERT OPINION:
The next 10 to 20 years will see a revolution in medicine and the life sciences that will change the elderly forever. It can only be compared to the current explosion of computing power and communication.
— *David A. Kekich, Maximum Life Foundation*

---

rganic milk from grass-fed cows has 67 percent more overall antioxidant and vitamin content than non-organic commercial milk, according to British researchers.

It takes 21 days to form a new habit or to break an old one, according to Dr. Maxwell Maltz in "Psycho-Cybernetics."

Don't mix coffee and other caffeinated beverages with iron-fortified breakfast cereal. The polyphenols (antioxidants) in coffee inhibit the absorption of iron by as much as 94 percent.

According to the United States Department of Agriculture (USDA) estimates, the average American consumes 3.3 pounds of spices a year.

One study shows that consuming less than a quarter teaspoon daily of cinnamon reduced blood sugar in people with diabetes by about 20 percent.

Chewing cinnamon gum improves attention and memory.

People who consume plenty of dairy products are less likely to develop gum disease, probably due to the lactic acid, according to Japanese researchers.

People who use pedometers walk an extra mile a day compared with those who don't use them, says the Journal of the American Medical Association.

The average person sheds 100 hairs a day.

WebMD.com reports that 75 to 90 percent of all doctor's visits are due to stress-related ailments and complaints.

In a study of 133 heavy smokers who were exposed to DNA damage from smoking, drinking four cups of decaffeinated green tea daily for four months reduced the signs of DNA damage by 31 percent.

15

EXPERT OPINION:

"The most important thing for people to know is that they now have some choices in health care, which allow better quality of life. These become pertinent since we're not living to 60 or 65. We could be living to 90 or 100."

— *Sangeeta Pati, M.D.*

According to Richard Schulze, N.D., "The large intestine is so big, that it is connected to, touches, sits next to or is in the vicinity of every major organ in the human body except the brain."

Studies show that people who are happily married live longer and healthier lives than single people.

Recent research studies reveal the antioxidants in tea may inhibit the growth of cancer cells and support cardiovascular health, according to Jeffrey Blumberg, Ph.D., F.A.C.N., professor and associate director of the Antioxidants Research Laboratory at the Jean Mayer USDA Human Nutrition Research Center on Aging at Tufts University.

Smokers who quit smoking before age 50 cut their risk of dying in the next 15 years in half, according to the National Conference of State Legislatures.

The scent of pink grapefruit can make men perceive women to be an average of six years younger than they really are, according to Dr. Alan Hirsch, director of The Smell & Taste Treatment and Research Foundation in Chicago. The world's first anti-aging perfume, Ageless, includes the essence of pink grapefruit and other scents. Studies show Ageless makes women look eight years younger to men.

Los Angeles-based Orly trademarked the term "Original French Manicure" in 1978.

Drowsy driving is responsible for at least 10,000 auto crashes, 71,000 injuries and 1,550 fatalities per year, according to the National Highway Traffic Safety Administration.

Investigators from the Howard Hughes Medical Institute (HHMI) have found that exercise improves learning and memory.

Iced tea was invented quite by accident at the 1904 St. Louis World's Fair. A young Englishman named Richard Blechynden, who had come all the way from India to bring teas from the Far East to the fair, sat idle in the heat while the other vendors prospered. Thinking quickly, he poured his tea over ice and it became an instant success.

Non-genetic hair loss is much worse in women who are deficient in iron and those who have low levels of the B vitamins. Nine out of 10 women aged 16 to 50 and one in three women over 50 are deficient in iron.

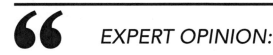 *EXPERT OPINION:*

The three hormones to address in mid-30s are: first, progesterone which, when out of balance, can contribute to lack of sleep, mood swings, anxiety and weight gain; second, thyroid; and third, melatonin.

— *Sangeeta Pati, M.D.*

Nearly four in 10 adults usually skip breakfast, what's been called "the most important meal of the day."

A report in the British journal The Lancet revealed that more than a quarter of Americans suffer daily pain.

According to a recent study, spending just 10 minutes talking to another person can improve your memory as well as your performance on tests.

Outside of human breast milk, coconut oil provides nature's most abundant source of lauric acid. Lauric acid is converted by the body into monolaurin, which has been show to inactivate viruses.

Research shows that organic fruit and vegetables contain as much as 40 percent more antioxidants, which are believed to help fend off cancer and heart disease.

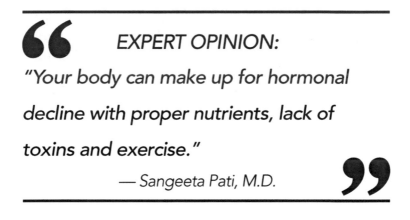

EXPERT OPINION:

"Your body can make up for hormonal decline with proper nutrients, lack of toxins and exercise."

— *Sangeeta Pati, M.D.*

Former Surgeon General Dr. Richard Carmona said in a 2006, 670-page study, "The debate is over. The science is clear. Secondhand smoke kills people."

Eating avocado can raise your HDL (good) cholesterol.

Nearly 10 percent of all adult men and 20 percent of all adult women are affected by varicose veins to some degree.

Studies have shown that women who drink green tea regularly have a lower incidence of breast cancer.

Cigarette smoking among adults in the U.S. is at its lowest level since Gallup began polling Americans about their smoking habits. Last year's figure showed 21 percent of U.S. adults smoked cigarettes, compared to 41 percent who reported smoking in 1944.

The British Medical Journal reported that close ties with children and other family members apparently have no impact on longevity, but those who have a very strong personal network of close friends and confidants show much higher survival rates.

According to Dr. Alan Hirsch, founder and neurological director of the Smell & Taste Treatment and Research Foundation in Chicago, breathing in the scent of peppermint will make you "more awake and alert, and that leads to feeling upbeat."

Studies have shown that one's health can improve when actively and personally engaged in helping others.

Chapter 3

Aging Backwards Escapades: Short Stories

It's In The Jeans

Years ago, around the time low-rise, bell-bottom jeans were first coming back in style and being worn by teenagers and "hip" fashionistas, I was still wearing my trusty, high-waisted, boot-cut Guess jeans. Guess jeans were expensive, so what was I going to do, throw them away? I didn't even wear jeans very often; I was into wearing skirts at the time. One day, my son asked me to take him to the smoothie shop for his favorite strawberry-banana concoction. I threw on a pair of my regular, old jeans and a sweatshirt and off we went. Smart enough to wait until he had his smoothie in hand, my son blurted out on the way back to the car, "Mom, please don't wear those jeans anymore, they make you look old."

That's all I had to hear. The next day I was in the dressing room at Nordstrom with my "personal shopper," trying on every pair of low-rise jeans in the store. What makes this story interesting is not the fact that I was behind the times or embarrassing my son, or even that I "looked old." What makes it interesting is that while I was in the dressing area, I met another woman who was around 50 years old, also shopping for low-rise jeans. She confided in me that her husband told her that if she, "... didn't go out and buy some 'young, hip-hugging' jeans, he planned to find a younger girl-friend." Of course, she knew he was joking, but yet, there she was in the dressing room at Nordstrom, trying to look young and hip in new jeans.

Lip Service

As the "anti-aging petri dish," I like to try all the latest products and innovations so I can tell everyone what works and what doesn't. People always send me products for review and I try to be fair and at least test them out. I once received a box of lip plumpers that sat in my kitchen for a while, so out of guilt or curiosity, I decided to try the product one morning right before my weekly radio show on Mix 100.7 Nancy & Chris Mornings. I smoothed the plumper onto my lips as directed at about 6 a.m. and left for the radio station. By the time I arrived 30 minutes later, I couldn't feel my tongue. My lips were plump, alright, but if I can't feel my tongue I can't really say, "This is a great product!"

At some point in the show, the brilliant and hilarious radio personality Nancy Alexander and I got to talking about this particular lip plumper on the air, commenting about the lack of feeling in my tongue. I told everyone that I wouldn't say the name because I felt I could not endorse this product with the peculiar side effect. Within one minute, every phone line lit up and we continued to get calls begging for the name of the product. We must have gotten dozens! Finally, to put a stop to all the calls, Nancy revealed the name of the product, which sold for a whopping $35 for a quarter of an ounce! I prefer to plump my lips naturally with Cynthia Rowland's Luscious Lips lip pump and keep my tongue intact. (See Jackie's Fancy chapter).

Gotta Potty? Well, That Depends ...
Back when liposuction was a huge surgery, I made an appointment to have the procedure done on my abdomen. Having experienced a C-section with the birth of my son, I thought it would be wise to plan ahead to minimize trips to the potty. I had a sudden flash of brilliance, or so I thought. "Why don't I buy Depends underwear for bladder control and use them while I recuperate?"
In theory, it sounded plausible. And this was before news broke of the NASA astronaut who allegedly drove 900 miles from Houston to Orlando wearing a diaper to avoid rest stops. I didn't want the checkout person at the store to think the Depends were for me, so I decided to buy Depends for men. "Maybe they'll think it's for my grandfather," I thought. Well, I can attest that Depends for men do not work for women. I should have figured as much, given the vast anatomical differences, but live and learn, right? Just another episode in Jackie's quest to keep Aging Backwards.

My Adventure as a Smurf
When I was in my late 30s, I decided to have a face peel. I did some research, talked to some people, asked around and settled on a peel with an interesting side effect: it turned your face blue. I didn't relish resembling a Smurf, but I was accustomed to sacrificing in the name of Aging Backwards. Over the years I've built up quite a threshold for pain, but I knew I was in trouble when I saw the portable fan being dragged out before

my procedure. The peel can only be done in a doctor's office, but his assistant was assigned to my case. She applied the acid in layers, using the fan to cool the burn in between passes.

It wasn't the worst pain I had ever experienced; it was somewhere between discomfort and agony. Since I did my research and was prepared to look un-usual, I had plenty of food in the house and cleared my calendar. The blue tint only lasted about 24 hours and then came what I call my "leather stage." You know how a baked potato skin looks after it's been in the oven too long? That sort of describes my face. Around the third day, the leather began to crack, then peel.

Of course, the doctor tells you not to peel your face, let it happen naturally, but with me that's akin to saying, "Just look at that chocolate and smell it, but don't eat it." At one point in the healing process, my skin was so taut that it actually pulled down my lower eyelids, giving me a freakish appearance. Wouldn't you know it, that day I had an emergency and had to run to the grocery store. The checkout girl didn't even try to hide her astonishment at my appearance and blurted out, "What happened to you?" I told her I had been caught in a fire, just to see her reaction. After about 10 days, my face had completely peeled, reveal-ing the most beautiful, pink, healthy skin I had ever seen. It looked beautiful for a while, but unfortunately it wasn't a permanent solution.

Community Service Fun — Bingo Anyone?

Many schools in Florida require students to fulfill a certain number of community service hours. I happen to feel that required community service is an oxymoron and I oppose it, but I'm not in charge of the program. My son opted to volunteer at the local independent living facility for bingo night. Since he was still too young to drive, I drove him there and played along. "That was fun," I told my son on the way home. "I'm going to volunteer at bingo every Monday night." Lead by example, right?

So the next day I called the activities director and asked if she would like a weekly volunteer for Monday night bingo. Her answer? A resounding "yes." I started calling the bingo numbers every Monday night and I'm still there. A friend of mine who was visiting from Houston invited me for drinks and dinner one Monday night. I asked him if he'd like to hang out with me at bingo and he said, "Why not?" I warned him not to win — the money is for the residents. Well, I guess my friend Jimmy is just a natural-born winner. He won three out of seven games. Each time he won, I glared at him from the front of the room and sent him telepathic thoughts: "Jimmy, what on earth are you doing?" You could feel the atmosphere in the room getting frostier each time he called out, "Bingo!" On the last game, Jimmy put all his winnings into the final pot, which was won by Frances. She was the only happy one in the room. To this day, the bingo ladies still ask about Jimmy (I guess they've forgiven him), and he still promises to come back and show them how to win.

Fraud Doctor

A friend and I decided to visit a California plastic surgeon for a consultation. Another friend of ours recommended him because, being out in Camarillo, he was much cheaper than a comparable Beverly Hills doctor. Plus, he didn't charge for consults. We weren't seriously considering having anything done, we just thought it would be a fun road trip from Los Angeles and an interesting experience. At the time, I was about 45 and she was 42, but she put down 37 on the forms we filled out. We went in together, and she was the first one in the chair. He looked at her file, took a cursory look at her and told her she didn't need a thing. He said she was still young and perhaps a little Botox was all she needed. It's true, she didn't need anything, but if she had any area that was beginning to show her age it was her neck, which is usually the first place to show age for many people. I was next in the chair.

The doctor looked at my chart and launched into a discourse that almost rivaled Lincoln's Gettysburg Address about how he could give me a neck lift and get rid of "all this," as he gestured under his chin. What's amazing about this is I had already had a neck lift at age 38, and my neck has been compared to that of a teenager by some of the doctors I know. My friend and I were both in such shock that we were rendered speechless. We walked out of the doctor's office and to this day we laugh about the fraud doctor who wanted to give me a neck lift with my teenage neck. So, watch out for anti-aging "specialists" who just want to take your money and aren't really going to do anything for you.

Smile, You're On Camera

Like many people of my generation, I went through life with the discoloration of tetracycline-stained teeth, which results from the antibiotic being introduced while the teeth are forming. With every "open wide" from every dentist I've ever seen, the first words I heard were, "Oh, I see you have tetracycline teeth." I've spent a fortune trying every whitening method available in the dentist's office and at home, with very little improvement. By my late 40s, I resigned myself to smiling with my mouth closed. Since I'm a very smiley person, this wasn't easy. Being a TV correspondent, it's imperative to smile, so I thought I had perfected the art of smiling with no teeth.

I was wrong. I'd end my segments with, "I'm Jackie Silver and we're Aging Backwards," and a toothless smile. Rob, my cameraman, would say, "You look kind of sad at the end, do it again, only smile more." So I said, "I'm Jackie Silver and we're Aging Backwards," with a bigger toothless smile. We'd go through a few rounds of that and, finally, Rob would give up and say, "We got it." Then, I got my Lumineers, porcelain veneers that go right over your own teeth. I found the most wonderful dentist, Dr. Dana in Tampa, Fla., who transformed my smile from one I was embarrassed of to that of a Hollywood star! Now I smile all the time and when I say, "I'm Jackie Silver and we're Aging Backwards," with a big smile at the end, Rob is very satisfied, and so am I. You can see before/after pictures on my Web site, AgingBackwards.com.

Mistaken Identity

My son is an avid golfer, and I like riding around the golf course on the cart with him every now and then. I enjoy the natural surroundings, breathing the fresh air and getting my needed vitamin D from sun on my legs. One day, I was hanging out with him at the chipping range, wearing no makeup, capri pants, a T-shirt and flip flops. A few other people were chipping nearby, including a boy whose grandfather had come to watch him. The boy's father came up to me and said, "My father [the boy's grandfather] asked me if you were Trent's girlfriend." Considering that my son was 17 at the time (he's just 18 now), I'll take it as a sure sign that I'm Aging Backwards!

The Key to Longevity?

I have always loved a good workout, but I didn't like to waste time with trivial stuff like stretching. Did I say trivial? Oops! I got a "trivia" lesson a few years ago while on a trip to New York City. I was advised not to miss breakfast at Norma's in Le Parker Meridien Hotel on West 57th Street. To the right of me sat Geraldo Rivera, and to my left sat an elderly man and his companion, a young woman who turned out to be a gerontology researcher. We struck up a conversation, as I'm prone to do just about anywhere with almost anyone. I found myself chatting with none other than Bert Morrow, Olympic hurdling champion and star of a famous Chiquita banana TV commercial. Talk about Aging Backwards! Mr. Morrow started hurdling at age 69!

At some point in the conversation, I asked him, "What is the key to longevity?" He gave me a one-word answer: stretching. We talked for a while about stretching and other topics, but that one word hit me hard and has stayed with me. It's so simple yet so often overlooked. There are numerous benefits to stretching, such as increasing flexibility, lowering the risk of injury, boosting energy, decreasing stress, increasing blood and nutrient flow to tissues, increasing range of motion and improving posture. Stretching can lengthen muscles and give that lean, toned look. It is a great warm-up or cool-down that can prevent soreness and promote faster recovery.

Death By Tanning

My friends were raving to me about their spray-on tanning booth experiences a few years ago. They told me how great the booths were, how quick, how convenient, how wonderful their faux tans looked. I had a special occasion for which I wanted to look 10 pounds thinner in 10 minutes – ergo, spray tan. I walked into the nearest tanning salon and after watching a required video, I was all set to get sprayed. I asked the teenage girl who ran the place if she had any nose plugs, which I had seen in the video and thought, "Good idea!" She didn't have any, nor did she have a towel I could put over my face, but she gave me a plastic shower cap and suggested I use it to shield my face. Apparently, no one ever warned her of the danger of suffocation from plastic. I took the shower cap anyway, just in case.

I proceeded to disrobe in the little dressing room and stepped into the booth with nothing but that shower cap. Suddenly, noxious fumes started spraying all around me and I began gasping for air. I tried the door, but amazingly, found myself locked in! Instinct forced me to put the shower cap to my face, so instead of suffocating from the tanning spray, I was now suffocating from plastic. My only recourse was to hold my breath, which I did for at least a minute while

I struggled with the door. Finally, the door flung open and I collapsed on the floor outside the booth gasping for air. Believe it or not, I was so mortified from the whole experience that I didn't ask for my money back and didn't even tell the teenage girl about my experience. I thought I was some sort of "tanning booth wimp" and she would simply laugh every time she repeated the story of the "crazy lady who almost suffocated in the tanning booth."

Needless to say, I've never tried one of those automatic spray tans again, but I have had beautiful spray tans applied by reputable aestheticians in salons.

This Really Bugged Me ...

About 10 years ago, I decided to try yoga, before it became mainstream. I thought, "I'll become more flexible, I'll reduce stress – I've even heard you can get taller." After much research, I joined a serene yoga studio in a beautiful stilt house nestled in the trees of a quiet neighborhood. The staff was very Zen-like and I just loved the ambience. Back then, most people didn't have their own yoga mats. You couldn't just pop into Target and buy one. So I used the yoga mats provided by the studio.

As is typical when you first start a new hobby or activity, I was very gung-ho and signed up for a three-month package that allowed me to attend three classes a week. I went faithfully Monday, Wednesday and Friday for a couple of weeks. I was thoroughly enjoying the experience, feeling less stressed and becoming more flexible.

During the first week, I noticed a couple of itchy bumps on my left shin, which would not go away. Finally, I decided to see a dermatologist, who informed me that I had scabies! Mistakenly considered a sexually transmitted disease, in reality it can be contracted through any skin-to-skin contact. Around the same time, I received a letter from my son's second-grade teacher announcing that scabies was discovered in the class. I volunteered regularly to read aloud to the children, which usually accompanied hugs from some of the students.

I felt I had a moral obligation to call the yoga studio, inform them of my condition and let them know I used many – if not all – of their yoga mats. I wasn't sure if scabies could be transferred through yoga mats, but I wasn't taking any chances of infecting other people.

"Hi, this is Jackie. I regret to tell you that I've been diagnosed with scabies, a highly contagious condition, and I have been using your yoga mats," I told the studio owner by phone. Well, she sure dropped that Zen demeanor pretty quickly when she practically shouted into the phone, "What?! Now I'll have to call every one of our students." She was horrified, and so was I. As you can imagine, I never showed my face again at the yoga studio and I was even too embarrassed to ask for a refund for the remaining classes.

Before being diagnosed, I ended up passing on my little eight-legged parasites to a friend of mine with whom I played Scrabble weekly. She, in turn, passed it on to her nail tech, who passed it on to her boyfriend who had a broken arm in a cast. He had to have the cast cut off because the scabies burrowed inside. Last I heard, they had broken up. Gee, I wonder why?

Chipmunk Cheeks Are Attractive ...
On the Chipmunk

In an effort to keep Aging Backwards, I visited one of my guru doctors, Roger Y. Murray, M.D. in Orlando, for a little rejuvenation. I explained that I wanted some Botox and Restylane injections. Dr. Murray agreed I could use a little pick-me-up with Botox and Restylane, but there was something he could do first to make a big difference that had nothing to do with those injectables. He pointed out, in the nicest way of course, that I had some jowls starting to form and he could "melt" the fat in my jaw line with some quick injections.

"Go for it," I exclaimed. If Dr. Murray suggests something to me, I listen. He knows me, he knows anti-aging, he's a medical doctor and he's an artist. All of my criteria are met. I forgot to mention to him that I was leaving in a couple of days to fly to Los Angeles for some important voice over auditions. He forgot to mention that I would look like a chipmunk for a few days – or maybe he mentioned it and I forgot to listen. I did fly to Los Angeles with my fat jaw, hoping nobody would notice. I mean, even if anyone noticed, people are too polite to ask about it, right? Wrong! Everyone asked me about it, including total strangers. Someone asked me if I had had my wisdom teeth extracted. Great excuse! That was my line for the next few days. By the way, Dr. Murray was right. My jowls melted and disappeared, taking years off my look.

Sometimes It Doesn't Pay to Eat Your Veggies

I don't get sick very often, but I was suffering from a very bad cold a few years ago while living in Los Angeles. In an effort to avoid a visit to the doctor's office, I elected to try the old standby: chicken soup. Not just any chicken soup, but my favorite Thai recipe – chicken lemongrass soup from a cute restaurant near Beverly Hills, which offered home delivery. I'd eaten this soup at least a dozen times before and I knew the ingredients: chicken broth, white meat chicken, mushrooms, coconut milk and lemongrass - soothing. This time, I noticed a green bean in the soup and thought, "Yeah, there should be more green vegetables in this soup." I ate it and to my utter astonishment, it was not a green bean, but the hottest chili pepper I had ever tasted. I was forced to put ice on my tongue for about an hour after that and even considered going to the hospital. My sinuses sure cleared up in a hurry, though.

Chapter 4

Aging Backwards Nutrition:
Eat, Drink & Be Young

We all know a balanced diet in the proper portions is crucial to good health, but sometimes "knowing" and "doing" can be two different things. I have simplified my nutritional plan down to its easiest form. I super-size my veggies and half-size everything else. Taking the emphasis off worrying, measuring, weighing and counting allows me to enjoy my food more and eat less.

 EXPERT OPINION:

Eat a little protein with every meal.
– Stephen T. Sinatra, M.D.

Gaining More Than Just Friendship

It's fun to dine out with friends, but keep these statistics in mind when you do: On average, if you dine with one other person, you will eat about 35 percent more than if you were alone. If you eat with a party of seven or more people, you will consume a whopping 95 percent more, or nearly twice as much as you would if you were eating alone. If you're at a table for four, you'll end up eating about 75 percent more calories than if you dined alone.

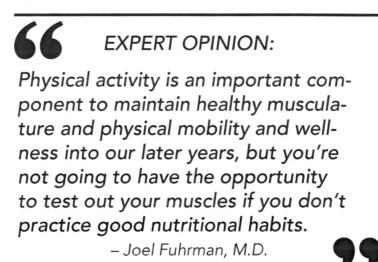

" EXPERT OPINION:

Physical activity is an important component to maintain healthy musculature and physical mobility and wellness into our later years, but you're not going to have the opportunity to test out your muscles if you don't practice good nutritional habits.
– Joel Fuhrman, M.D. **"**

Not-Too-Sweet News

Experts believe a lifetime of overeating sugar can cause wrinkles. A natural process called glycation is the culprit. With glycation, sugar in your bloodstream attaches to proteins to form harmful new molecules called "advanced glycation end products," or AGEs, appropriately. The more sugar you eat, the more AGEs you develop. The more ages you develop, the more they damage adjacent proteins in a domino-like fashion, according to Fredric Brandt, M.D., a dermatologist and author of "10 Minutes 10 Years." Besides damaging collagen, a high-sugar diet also affects the type of collagen you have – another factor in how resistant skin is to wrinkling. The most abundant collagen types in the skin are I, II and III, with type III being the most stable and long-lasting. Glycation turns type III collagen into type I, which is more fragile, making the skin look and feel less supple. It also leaves you more vulnerable to sun damage. Diabetics can have up to 50 times the number of AGEs in their skin than non-diabetics. That's another good reason to cut out sugar and super-size your veggies.

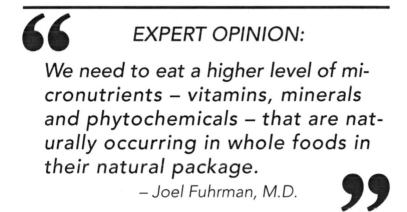

EXPERT OPINION:

We need to eat a higher level of micronutrients – vitamins, minerals and phytochemicals – that are naturally occurring in whole foods in their natural package.
– Joel Fuhrman, M.D.

Go Organic

A study into organic food has found that it is more nutritious than ordinary produce and may help to lengthen people's lives. The research project, with a price tag of $24 million, showed that organic fruits and vegetables contain as much as 40 percent more antioxidants, which are believed to help fend off cancer and heart disease. They also contain more beneficial minerals such as iron and zinc, the Sunday Times reported.

Researchers grew fruit and vegetables and raised cattle on adjacent organic and non-organic sites on a 725-acre farm attached to Newcastle University and at other sites in Europe. They found that levels of antioxidants in milk from organic herds were up to 90 percent higher than those from conventional herds.

Organic tomatoes from Greece were also found to have significantly higher levels of antioxidants. Professor Carlo Leifert, coordinator of the four-year project, said the differences were so marked that organic produce could help increase the nutrient intake of those people not eating the recommended five portions a day of fruit and vegetables.

---

66 *EXPERT OPINION:*

The body is a finely-tuned machine. We just have to get rid of toxic hunger and not eat recreationally and not eat because we're food addicts, rather we have to eat when we really have the desire through true hunger.
– *Joel Fuhrman, M.D.*

Let's Do Lunch

Salad can be an excellent food choice because you can combine plenty of vegetables with protein for a nutritious meal. Use the dark-green, leafy lettuces instead of iceberg lettuce for your base. Then, add taste and antioxidants to your salad by going for the reds. Make sure to add in plenty of red veggies and fruits, such as tomatoes, beets, red peppers, radicchio, red cabbage, apples and strawberries.

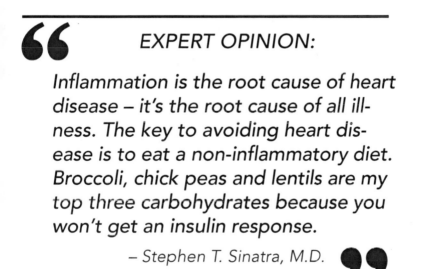

EXPERT OPINION:

Inflammation is the root cause of heart disease – it's the root cause of all illness. The key to avoiding heart disease is to eat a non-inflammatory diet. Broccoli, chick peas and lentils are my top three carbohydrates because you won't get an insulin response.

– Stephen T. Sinatra, M.D.

A Little Goes a Long Way

If you like creamy salad dressings, here's a way to enjoy them more while using less. Thin your salad dressing with fresh-squeezed lemon juice and a dash of olive oil. I love the creamy salad dressings, even though I know they're not the healthiest choice, so here's what I do: I buy a light but heavily flavored salad dressing like an organic Caesar light. I pour some of the creamy dressing in a bowl, and then thin it with fresh-squeezed lemon juice and just a touch of extra virgin olive oil. Not only does it taste yummy, it cuts the amount of the creamy dressing I use in half, thus cutting the fat in half, and also allows the dressing to spread more evenly on my salad.

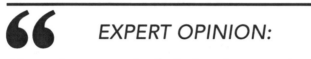

EXPERT OPINION:

True hunger is felt in the neck or the throat, not in the stomach or the head. One of the benefits of throat hunger is that you get a tremendous 50 percent increase in the ability to taste the flavor of the food. Natural foods taste better when you're really hungry.

– Joel Fuhrman, M.D.

Big Flavor, Small Portion

Try my crouton trick. I buy a bag of the most flavorful, whole-grain croutons I can find – something very garlicky. Then I pour the croutons into a big zipper baggy, take out my meat mallet and start hammering away. I crush the croutons to the point where they are very small crumbs, about the size of Grape

Nuts cereal. (By the way, this doubles as a great stress reducer!). Once your salad is tossed with your lemon juice/creamy dressing mixture, spoon a teaspoon or two of crouton crumbs over the top for a zing of extra flavor with practically no added calories or fat.

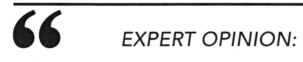

EXPERT OPINION:

There are a lot of health benefits associated with eating coconut oil, but there's always a fear people have that it's going to promote heart disease – that's not true.

– Bruce Fife, C.N., N.D.

Go Nuts!

Add a small amount of raw nuts to your salad for extra crunch and nutrients. Raw, unsalted nuts are good for your health because they're high in fiber and they contain monounsaturated fats, which help to lower bad cholesterol (LDL) and raise good cholesterol (HDL). Pumpkin seeds are a rich source of vitamins A, B1, B2, B3, calcium, iron and even a small amount of protein. Sesame seeds are considered one of the highest sources of calcium in the world when the husks are intact (dark brown in color). Find them at your local health food store. Walnuts are the only nuts that contain a significant amount of omega-3 fatty acids, essential for good health.

> **EXPECT OPINION:**
>
> *Most hot flashes are associated with women who eat a very high preserved food diet. Women who eat natural diets don't tend to get hot flashes.*
>
> *– Roger Y. Murray, M.D.*

EXPERT OPINION:

Most hot flashes are associated with women who eat a very high preserved food diet. Women who eat natural diets don't tend to get hot flashes.

– Roger Y. Murray, M.D.

The Odiferous Onion

Don't be put off by its pungent aroma – the onion is an excellent source of nutrients. Onions are also low in calories with only 30 per serving. They're sodium-, fat- and cholesterol-free and provide fiber, vitamin C, vitamin B6, potassium and other key nutrients. Research shows that getting five daily servings of fruit and veggies may help guard against certain illnesses, so chop up some onion with your next salad. That's nothing to cry about!

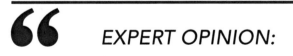

EXPERT OPINION:

I would consider eggs the cleanest, least polluted source of animal protein.

– Joel Fuhrman, M. D.

Get Your Protein Right Here

    Eggs are an "eggcellent" source of protein.
Here are some eggy facts:
• The average egg-laying hen lays 257 eggs per year.
• To prevent the yolk of a hard-boiled egg from getting a green ring, cook the eggs more gently. Boiling also makes them hard and rubbery, so cook on low to medium heat.
• There is no nutritional difference between brown eggs and white eggs.
• Contrary to popular belief, blood spots found on egg yolks do not mean the egg has been fertilized. They are caused by the rupture of a blood vessel on the yolk during the formation of the egg.
• Based on the essential amino acids it provides, egg protein is second only to mother's milk for human nutrition, according to the Iowa Egg Council.
• A large egg has 75 calories; extra-large has 84 calories.

 EXPERT OPINION:

All the studies on aging show that when we eat fewer calories, we slow the metabolic rate. Our bodies and our tissues age more slowly if our metabolic rate and body temperature are lower.

– *Joel Fuhrman, M.D.*

Chocoholics' Choice

Okay, chocoholics, here's the best news ever! According to new research, eating a small amount of dark chocolate every day can thin the blood and cut the risk of clots in much the same way that taking aspirin does! Hurray! Researchers have known for almost 20 years that dark chocolate can lower blood pressure and has other beneficial effects on blood flow. But new research suggests two tablespoons of dark chocolate a day is enough to have a beneficial effect and cut the risk of clots, according to research professor Diane Becker of Johns Hopkins University.

Chocolate Tap Water?

Coming soon – chocolate toothpaste and chocolate water? It may not be as fanciful as it sounds. According to Arman Sadeghpour, who holds a doctorate from Tulane University, an extract of cocoa powder that occurs naturally in chocolate, teas and some other foods might be an effective, natural alternative to fluoride. In fact, his research revealed that cocoa was even more effective than fluoride at fighting cavities. The extract – a white crystalline powder whose chemical makeup is similar to that of caffeine – helps harden tooth enamel and makes the teeth less susceptible to decay. The cocoa extract could offer the first major innovation in toothpaste manufacturing since fluoride was added in 1914.

As with many studies, it's been tested on animals and is still years away from human use. But hey, chocolate toothpaste and chocolate water would be worth waiting for, in my humble opinion.

EXPERT OPINION:
Even in middle age, adopting a
healthy lifestyle can lower the risk for
heart disease and premature death.

– *Ray Sahelian, M.D.*

Cut It Out

Renowned neurosurgeon and author, Russell L. Blaylock, M.D., stresses that it is important to avoid excitotoxins in food. These include monosodium glutamate (MSG), aspartame, hydrolyzed proteins, isolated proteins, vegetable protein, soy protein isolates, soy protein, soy milk, natural flavoring, sodium or calcium caseinate and others. According to Dr. Blaylock, all of these food additives worsen brain excitation and have been shown to specifically target the amygdala nucleus – a set of neurons in the brain's temporal lobe, which can lead to brain dysfunction.

In another study, Peter Piper (his real name), a professor of molecular biology and biotechnology at Sheffield University in the U.K., warns us to avoid the preservative sodium benzoate, found in some soft drinks, many pickled products and certain salad dressings and prepared foods, to name a few. Don't be fooled by the professor's "cute" name, there's nothing funny about the effects of sodium benzoate.

According to Professor Piper, the preservative inactivates the mitochondria, or energy center, of the body's DNA. "The mitochondria consumes the oxygen to give you energy and if you damage it - as happens in a number of diseased states - then the cell starts to malfunction very seriously. And there is a whole array of diseases that are now being tied to damage to this DNA — Parkinson's and quite a lot of neurodegenerative diseases, but above all the whole process of aging," said Professor Piper.

 EXPERT OPINION:

Changing our diet back to our more natural diet and not eating refined, processed carbohydrates could help lead to aging backwards.

– Al Sears, M.D.

Drink To Your Health

The good news about coffee just keeps on coming. Experts from the University of Scranton in Pennsylvania have told us, "Coffee has more antioxidants than any food or drink in the American diet." Finnish researchers told us that people who drank at least three to four cups of coffee a day had a nearly 30 percent lower risk of developing type 2 diabetes. The American Academy of Neurology told us that women 65 and older can protect their memories by drinking three cups of coffee a day. The Harvard School of Public Health says drinking up to six cups of coffee a day may keep us from dying prematurely because it cuts the risk of dying from heart disease. Anyone want to join me for a coffee break?

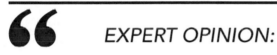 *EXPERT OPINION:*

Drinking a reasonable amount of water by a healthy person, such as about four to six glasses a day rather than eight, is enough to flush out toxins. As to skin, drinking lots of water does not necessarily increase the water content of the skin.

– Ray Sahelian, M.D.

Salud!

Red wine and red grapes contain a chemical called resveratrol that can offset some of the effects of overeating. It won't make you lose weight, but can possibly help you become as healthy as a normal-weight person, lowering glucose levels, improving your heart and helping your liver. Scientists fed lab rats a diet that was 60 percent fat, which led to obese rats with insulin resistance and cardiovascular disease. Then they divided them into two groups and continued to feed them the 60 percent fat diet, but one group also got resveratrol. The rats receiving resveratrol had lower glucose levels and their hearts and livers became healthier, plus they were sprier than the other group.

Even though they didn't lose any weight, their health became as good as a rat on a normal diet. The rats on the non-resveratrol diet had shorter life spans, but the overweight resveratrol group lived as long as rats on a normal diet. The scientists believe resveratrol may activate SIRT1, a gene associated with longevity. So, I'd like to offer a toast to longevity with red wine ... in moderation, of course.

EXPERT OPINION:
Use detoxification measures in your life at all times. Toxicity is a major factor in aging – be aware of chemicals, xenoestrogens, petrochemicals, perfumes you put on your skin, insecticides, pesticides, radiation, PCBs, chlorine ... We live in a sea of chemicals.

– Stephen T. Sinatra, M.D.

Tea Time

Many recent studies and reports have attributed health benefits to tea, especially green tea. "Fruits, vegetables and tea all contain important antioxidants," according to Jeffrey Blumberg, Ph.D., F.A.C.N., chief of the Antioxidants Research Laboratory at the Jean Mayer USDA Human Nutrition Research Center on Aging at Tufts University. "Research suggests these phytonutrients may contribute substantially to the promotion of health and the prevention of chronic disease. For example, recent research studies reveal the antioxidants in tea may inhibit the growth of cancer cells and support cardiovascular health."

Contrary to what many people believe, both green and black tea have about the same amount of caffeine, since both teas are derived from the same plant — the Camelia sinensis — and only the processing differs. If you brew the green tea for a shorter amount of time, which is recommended, it will have a lower caffeine content. Otherwise, the raw teas are nearly identical.

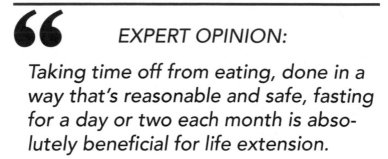

EXPERT OPINION:

Taking time off from eating, done in a way that's reasonable and safe, fasting for a day or two each month is absolutely beneficial for life extension.

– *Joel Fuhrman, M.D.*

Chapter 5

Aging Backwards Supplements:
To B12 or Not to B12 ...

  EXPERT OPINION:

There is currently no evidence that taking supplements or hormones (such as human growth hormone) will make us live longer. However, it seems reasonably safe to take small amounts of certain supplements that have shown in preliminary research to be helpful.

– Ray Sahelian, M.D.

ost doctors agree that our bodies need vitamins and minerals to function properly, but some doctors, such as Mallika Marshall, M.D. of Chelsea, Mass., maintain that the

average healthy American can get all the nutrients necessary by eating a balanced diet that includes five servings
of vegetables and fruit daily.

In fact, two studies debunk the theory that
taking B vitamins to reduce levels of an amino acid
in blood called homocysteine could protect against
heart attacks and strokes. The studies did show that
the vitamins reduced the homocysteine levels, but that
reduction failed to translate into a reduction in heart
attacks and strokes. The studies were conducted by
teams at McMaster University in Canada and the University of Tromso in Norway and were reported in the
New England Journal of Medicine. One wrinkle in the
results was that the findings pertained to people with
heart disease.

Annette Dickinson, a representative from The
Council for Responsible Nutrition, a trade group that
represents supplement makers, had this to say about
the findings: "These studies did not test whether B
vitamins used by healthy people can help keep them
healthy. Instead, they looked at whether B vitamins can
treat or reverse heart disease in people who already
have it. Vitamins should not be expected to perform
like drugs — their greatest promise is in prevention."

---

66 *EXPERT OPINION:*

People think that a longevity secret is to take as many antioxidants as possible in high doses, but more is not necessarily better.

– *Ray Sahelian, M.D.*

By now you've probably heard of antioxidants and their beneficial role in fighting free radical damage in our bodies, which has been linked to many diseases as well as aging. In case you've ever wondered who figured all that out, the answer is Dr. Denham Harman. He proposed the free radical theory of aging in 1955. There are many supplements on the market today that act as antioxidants, not to mention some foods that are natural sources, such as blueberries and green tea.

The supplements listed below are commonly referred to as having anti-aging properties and this is just a tiny sampling of what's out there. But as always, you should consult with your doctor before starting any type of supplementation and obtain proper dosing instructions.

Acetyl-L-Carnitine

Acetyl-l-carnitine (also called carnitine and L-carnitine) helps the body convert fatty acids into energy, which is used primarily by the muscles throughout the body. Our bodies produce carnitine in the liver and kidneys and store it in the skeletal muscles, heart, brain and sperm. There can be many causes for carnitine deficiency, including a high-fat diet, genetic factors and certain medications. Some studies have shown that people who took carnitine supplements significantly lowered their total cholesterol and triglycerides, and increased their HDL (healthy) cholesterol levels.

Alpha-Lipoic Acid

Also called ALA, alpha-lipoic acid is present in meats, spinach, broccoli and potatoes. Its primary function is to produce glutathione, which is responsible for dissolving toxins in the liver. ALA also neutralizes free radicals in our body resulting from tobacco smoke, car exhaust, deep-fried foods and alcohol, to name a few. The subject of intensive research, this may be the most important antioxidant of all in protecting the brain and neurological tissues from damage. Alpha-lipoic acid has the unique ability to pass into the brain, where is helps with regeneration of other antioxidants, such as vitamin C and E and glutathione. In addition to the supplement form, ALA is also found in some cosmetic creams as an antioxidant to prevent wrinkles.

>   *EXPERT OPINION:*
>
> *For those who are not able to stop their smoking habit, it would seem that taking vitamin C partially mitigates the harm caused to the blood vessels. A dose of 200 to 500 mg of vitamin C taken once or twice a day seems reasonable.*
>
> — *Ray Sahelian, M.D.*

Coenzyme-Q-10

This vitamin-like substance (also known as ubiquinone) was discovered in 1957. Commonly called CoQ10, it is present in most red blood cells and is responsible for the body's own production of energy. Scientific studies have linked it to a stronger immune system, lower blood pressure and slower aging. Studies in mice shows it increases their life span by 25 percent. CoQ10 is found in all cells, where it is responsible for manufacturing ATP, the basic energy molecule. Organs such as the liver and heart, which require the most energy, have the highest concentrations of CoQ10.

Curcumin

Curcumin has been hailed as an extremely powerful brain protector. A study in the journal Experimental Neurology found that curcumin dramatically improved synaptic plasticity and mental ability, and reduced free radicals in animals with severe brain injuries.

D-Ribose

Ribose is a type of sugar normally made in the body from glucose and provides every cell in the body with energy. Athletes take it to increase stamina and endurance and help them to recover from workouts more quickly. The theory is that ribose helps by supplying cells in the muscle tissue with a continuous supply of energy.

Garlic

Garlic has been used medicinally for at least 3,000 years. Many people have viewed its benefits as merely folklore until medical studies proved that garlic could lower cholesterol, prevent blood clots, prevent cancer and reduce blood pressure. Garlic contains more than 100 biologically useful chemicals whose benefits have been reported on in more than 1,000 scientific studies, according to the American Medical Association. If you don't want to go around smelling like a giant garlic clove, you can get the health benefits of garlic by taking it in supplement form. Adesh K. Jain, M.D., of the Clinical Research Center and Tulane University School of Medicine in New Orleans, conducted a 12-week study in which 20 men and women were given 900 milligrams of garlic powder tablets daily and 22 people were given a placebo.

By the end of the study, total blood cholesterol levels dropped by an average of six percent among those taking the tablets, compared to only a one percent drop among the placebo group. The people who took the garlic tablets also showed an 11 percent decrease in LDL cholesterol, compared with a 3 percent drop in the placebo group.

Grape Seed Extract

Grape seed extract is a powerful antioxidant and anti-inflammatory that has been shown to effectively strengthen the walls of blood vessels, which may help prevent aneurysms, strokes and heart attacks. Smoking severely weakens the walls of blood vessels and taking grape seed extract has been shown to counteract this effectively.

L-Carnosine

This is highly concentrated in skeletal muscles, heart muscle and brain tissue. According to reports, carnosine has the remarkable ability to rejuvenate cells approaching the end of their life cycle. As an antioxidant, carnosine effectively helps to neutralize the most destructive free radicals. Unlike most antioxidants, which work by prevention, carnosine protects after free radicals have been released. Carnosine has been shown to block the decay of protein function, called glycosylation. It also blocks amyloid production, the substance found in the brains of Alzheimer's patients. Plus, it's been credited with anti-cancer and immune-boosting effects.

Magnesium

Magnesium has been shown to improve heart function and increase blood flow through the coronary arteries. In case of a heart attack, it can significantly reduce the severity of damage to the heart muscle. According to research, it can also reduce the risk of heart disease, stroke and type 2 diabetes.

Omega-3 (EPA and DHA)

Omega-3 essential fatty acids (EFAs) are polyunsaturated "good" fats found in the oil of cold-water fish such as salmon, mackerel and tuna. Omega-3 EFAs help maintain good cholesterol and blood pressure levels and strong heartbeat. While Omega-3s are important to the body's overall good health, they can't be made by the body and must be acquired through diet or supplementation. They may also help enhance skin, hair and mood.

 EXPERT OPINION:

Restore optimal function to your cells so that they do what they do best — keep you healthy happy, energetic, cancer-free, at your optimal weight and plaque-free.

— Sangeeta Pati, M.D.

Resveratrol

Resveratrol is an ingredient found in the skin and seeds of red grapes used to make red wine that seems to have heart-healthy benefits, including lowering blood pressure, reducing "bad" cholesterol and lowering the risk of developing blood clots. An even newer finding suggests that resveratrol may be the first line of defense against breast cancer. Lead author of the report, Eleanor G. Rogan, Ph.D., a professor at the Eppley Institute for Research in Cancer and Allied Diseases at the University of Nebraska Medical Center said, "Resveratrol has the ability to prevent the first step that occurs when estrogen starts the process that leads to cancer by blocking the formation of the estrogen DNA adducts. We believe that this could stop the whole progression that leads to breast cancer down the road."

The findings were reported in Cancer Prevention Research, the journal of the American Association for Cancer Research. Since alcohol should only be consumed in moderation and some people cannot have any alcohol, scientists have created resveratrol supplements to provide all the benefits without the alcohol.

S-Adenosylmethionine (SAMe)

SAMe occurs naturally in the body and is widely distributed in the tissues of young, healthy adults. It plays a role in the immune system, maintains cell membranes and helps produce and break down brain chemicals. Many scientific studies indicate that SAMe may help in treating depression, fibromyalgia and osteoarthritis, since it reduces joint inflammation and promotes cartilage repair. It may also help to prevent or reverse liver damage due to alcohol misuse, viruses and pollution. In addition, SAMe may decrease the frequency, intensity and duration of headaches, as shown in a preliminary study.

Superoxide Dismutase (SOD)

Superoxide dismutase (SOD) is a powerful anti-oxidant that has been called an "anti-aging" substance by doctors and scientists. Oxygen, which gives us life, also gets converted inside our cells into free radical molecules or "oxidants" that damage our cells, resulting in what's called "oxidative stress." According to one estimate, oxidants bombard the DNA inside every one of our cells roughly 10,000 times a day. The same process that causes an apple to turn brown and metal to rust is also happening to us.

Conventional antioxidant supplements (such as vitamins A, C and E) are known as "consumable" antioxidants because as they neutralize free radicals they are consumed in the process. The body's natural antioxidant enzymes SOD and Catalase (CAT) each destroy up to 100,000 free radicals per second and continue to function for 24 hours, so they are literally thousands of times more powerful than conventional supplements.

Dr. Joe McCord, while a graduate doctoral student at Duke University, discovered superoxide dismutase more than 30 years ago. SOD has shown promise in fighting the oxidative stress that is linked to not only aging, but also major diseases such as cancer, heart disease, diabetes, Alzheimer's and arthritis.

Increasing SOD and CAT has been shown to slow aging and extend life. One supplement called

Protandim contains a unique combination of phytonutrients in a small supplement that clinical tests show increases the body's own production of SOD by 30 percent, increases the production of CAT by 50 percent and decreases the level of oxidative stress in people by 40 percent for "aging backwards at the cellular level." A single daily caplet of Protandim creates a cascade of your body's natural catalytic antioxidants that destroy millions of free radicals per second, on a continuous basis - 24/7. (See Jackie's Fancy chapter for Protandim).

" EXPERT OPINION:
I don't think we are going to find out about the risks and benefits of multivitamins until several different formulas, developed by experienced nutritional experts, are tested for at least 10 to 20 years on a large group of people.

– *Ray Sahelian, M.D.*

Vitamin D

A study from the Harvard School of Public Health published in the Journal of the American Medical Association suggests that for some people, having high levels of vitamin D in their blood might be linked to reducing the risk of developing Multiple Sclerosis (MS). "If confirmed, this finding suggests that many cases of MS could be prevented by increasing vitamin D levels," said Alberto Ascherio, associate professor of nutrition and epidemiology at Harvard School of Public Health.

The study found that among whites, the risk of developing MS significantly decreased with increasing levels of vitamin D in the blood. For people in the top 20 percent of vitamin D concentration, there was a 62 percent lower risk of MS compared to people with the lowest 20 percent concentration.

Multiple Sclerosis is a progressive, degenerative disease that affects the central nervous system. About 350,000 people in the US suffer from MS and another 2 million worldwide. It's more common in women than in men. Unlike other vitamins, the body can manufacture vitamin D with exposure to sunlight. Some foods rich in vitamin D include milk, eggs, shiitake mushrooms, cod liver oil and fatty fish. According to doctors, the best way to keep your Vitamin D levels optimal is to get 10 to 15 minutes a day of direct sunlight on three-quarters of your body.

EXPERT OPINION:
"Even though high dosages of calcium and vitamin D may help bones become stronger and reduce the risk for fractures, they could also potentially raise the risk of brain calcifications leading to mental decline."

— *Ray Sahelian, M.D.*

Chapter 6

Aging Backwards Exercise:
The Real Fountain of Youth?

When people hear the words "anti-aging," they tend to think of face creams or lasers or even plastic surgery, but there is a myriad of other aspects of "Aging Backwards." Exercise is quite possibly one of the most disliked — but it doesn't have to be!

 EXPERT OPINION:

"Exercise is all about change. If you do a static exercise program you'll get benefit for a couple of weeks, but then your body's already made the adaptive response."
— Al Sears, M.D.

I personally love to work out, but I know scores of people who consider exercise the bane of their existence. Many people are looking for shortcuts, magic pills or creams to keep them young, but the reality is it takes work. I consider exercise to be my magic pill. Not only does working out benefit the heart and lungs, increase strength and muscle tone and keep the body lean, but it also helps to lower stress levels, get rid of toxins and actually makes the skin look younger by increasing circulation and delivering nutrients to skin cells.

According to Audrey Kunin, M.D., a Kansas City, Mo. dermatologist and the author of "The DERMAdoctor Skinstruction Manual," another benefit of exercise is that it gives the skin optimum conditions for making collagen, the support fibers that help keep wrinkles and lines at bay.

Add Five Years

No matter how naturally thin a person is, he or she still needs to exercise to stay healthy. "Many people, especially slim people, believe that the only benefit that can be achieved from exercising is weight loss," said Dr. Gary O'Donovan, exercise physiologist at Brunel University in West London. "That is not the case. Our study suggests that slim people need to exercise as much as others in order to stay healthy and keep LDL cholesterol in check."

Dr. O'Donovan devised his study to see how exercise affected a person's health profile and he found that those who did well in fitness tests were likely to live around five years longer than those who were sedentary.

> **EXPERT OPINION:**
>
> *Human growth hormone is the closest we've ever found to an anti-aging 'elixir.' It reverses nearly every identifiable aspect of aging. We secrete a lot of it when we're young, less as we age. You can secrete growth hormone with short duration, higher intensity exercise.*
>
> — *Al Sears, M.D.*

More Exercise, Fewer Colds

According to data, the average adult may get two to five colds per year. When I first read that I was shocked because I only get a cold about every other year. Then I read the next part: the research team found that, of people who participated in a study including 547 healthy men and women between 20 and 70 (average age 48), the ones who had a moderate to high level of daily physical activity experienced 25 percent fewer colds than the people with low daily activity. During the fall months, that number jumped to 32 percent fewer upper respiratory infections. I knew my daily workouts were good for keeping my weight down, taking care of my heart and keeping depression away, but who knew they also keep me from getting sick?

The study also revealed that while moderate to high daily activity reduced the risk of illness, extremely high levels may have a negative effect on the immune system and could increase the risk of catching a cold. For example, running a marathon can deplete immune system defenses and actually make you more vulnerable to getting sick in the week after the race.

Think and Grow Thin
A recent study revealed that if you think you're getting the proper exercise, you could actually lose more weight doing the same activity as a person who thinks their activity level is too low to lose. Just another great example of "mind over matter." The study included hotel housekeepers who were divided into two groups. One group was told the calorie expenditure for various activities, such as changing linens for 15 minutes (40 calories burned), vacuuming for 15 minutes (50 calories burned) and cleaning bathrooms for 15 minutes (60 calories burned). The other group was told nothing about the health benefits of their daily chores.

After four weeks, the first group who had been told of the health benefits of their work had lost an average of two pounds, lowered their blood pressure by almost 10 percent and reduced their body fat by almost .5 percent. The other group experienced no noticeable changes in their weight, body or health. "The changes were a function of the change in mindset alone," said lead researcher Ellen Langer in an article published in Psychological Science.

> ❝
> *EXPERT OPINION:*
>
> *For someone who has type 2 diabetes, all attempts should be made to use diet, exercise, herbs and natural supplements before resorting to drugs.*
> — *Ray Sahelian, M.D.* ❞

Gimme Those Young Cells

I've been saying for years that I want to find out how to keep Aging Backwards at the cellular level. Well, I finally got my answer. According to an article in Newsweek magazine, exercise can help reverse the aging process at the genetic level. Thank goodness I never gave up on my workouts! According to the study, a group of 25 elderly volunteers aged 65 and older (average age 77) did one-hour sessions of strength training in a gym twice a week for six months using standard gym equipment and doing three sets of 10 reps for each muscle group. The researchers then compared cells from the thighs of the elderly group to thigh-muscle cells from a group of young people whose average age was 22.

The researchers were expecting the workouts to improve strength, but what they were not expecting were dramatic changes at the genetic level. Simon Melov, director of genomics at the Buck Institute in

Novato, Calif., and co-author of the study said, "The genetic fingerprint was reversed to that of younger people - not entirely, but enough to say that their genetic profile was more like that of young people than old people.

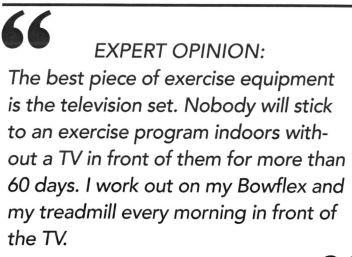

EXPERT OPINION:
The best piece of exercise equipment is the television set. Nobody will stick to an exercise program indoors without a TV in front of them for more than 60 days. I work out on my Bowflex and my treadmill every morning in front of the TV.

— Roger Y. Murray, M.D.

Buff Mice Burn Fat

Lifting weights could be as effective as endurance exercises, such as running, when it comes to burning fat and avoiding diabetes. A team from Boston University School of Medicine genetically engineered some mice to grow a specific type of muscle, called Type II, which develops as a result of resistance training. Type I muscle forms as a result of endurance training. Kenneth Walsh, one of the study's team members said, "We've shown that Type II muscle does more than allow you to pick up heavy objects. It's also important in controlling whole-body metabolism. If you have these muscles, even when you are not doing much, you are still burning up energy."

Buff Mice Fight Cancer

Just when you think there can't possibly be any more health benefits to exercise than the ones I've covered ad nauseam, here's one I hadn't heard before: exercise can even protect against skin cancer. Dr. Allan Conney, a Rutgers University cancer researcher, and his team tested some mice in two groups. One group of mice had an exercise wheel so they could "work out," while the other group of mice didn't have their own home gym. They exposed both groups of mice to UVB light — the type that can cause tumors — and found that the buff mice took longer to develop tumors and developed fewer and smaller tumors. Let me mention again that exercise is free. Anyone can do it, but check with your doctor if you have limitations.

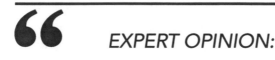

The PACE Program (Progressively Accelerating Cardiopulmonary Exertion) builds muscle at the same time it burns fat. With PACE, we push ourselves a little bit more with focus and progressive intensity, but then focus on the parasympathetic recovery, the relaxation response, where you rest in between and focus on lowering your heart rate with conscious intent.

— Al Sears, M.D.

Aging Backwards Exercise Tips
• Trick yourself into working out. If I'm feeling tired or sluggish and start to make excuses to myself about why I'm not going to work out, I put on my gym clothes and shoes and tell myself, "I'll just 'play along,' not really put any effort into it and then I'll at least feel better than if I just sat around." Five minutes into "playing along," I feel energized and I'm doing a full-blown workout, which I would have skipped altogether if I hadn't tricked myself into doing it.

• Get some cute workout clothes that make you feel great. If you like your exercise outfits and you feel good in them, it can mean the difference between working out and not working out, especially if you go to a gym. I like to exercise at home. I have a variety of fun and interesting DVDs that I like to work out to. The Firm workout is one of my all-time favorites.

These women are in the most fantastic shape! I don't know about you, but if my trainers look terrific, I feel confident and inspired by them, knowing I could look like them if I stick with the program. And it works. My body has definitely changed since starting The Firm. Even when I'm working out all alone at home, I make sure I'm wearing a cute workout outfit. It's all about doing it for me, not for anyone else.

• Use visualization to achieve the results you want. Many studies have shown that there is a powerful mind-body connection that can be beneficial in so many ways. What is the mind-body connection and how does it work? Can what we think actually have an effect on our bodies? According to research, it can.

Our psychological/emotional state affects the endocrine system. For example, when we experience fear, the hormone adrenaline is released into our systems. When we have no fear, there's no adrenaline flowing. The hypothalamus — the emotional center of the brain — transforms emotions into physical response, affecting appetite, body temperature, circulation and a host of other functions. The hypothalamus is the receptor for neuropeptides, chemical messenger hormones that carry emotions back and forth between the mind and body and influence the immune system in a big way.

Neuropeptides link perception in the brain to the body via hormones, organs and cellular activity so the mind and body work together as one unit.

66

EXPERT OPINION:

The best exercise you can do is the

one you will stick with.

— *Roger Y. Murray, M.D.* **99**

It's a Stretch
Don't like to "waste time" with stretching before and after a workout? There are numerous benefits to stretching, such as increasing flexibility, lowering the risk of injury, boosting energy, decreasing stress, increasing blood and nutrient flow to tissues, increasing range of motion and improving posture. Stretching can lengthen muscles and give that lean, toned look. It's a great warm-up or cool-down that can prevent soreness and promote faster recovery.

Tips for Stretching
• Warm up first. It's best to stretch after your muscles are warmed up, such as after a few minutes of low-intensity walking or other gentle movements. If you're short on time, try stretching immediately after a shower or even in a hot bath. The warm water will increase

muscle temperature enough to make the muscles more flexible. If you belong to a gym, check with the trainers for suggestions or ask your physician before starting any workout program.
• Try buddy stretching. When stretching with a friend, you can use each other for resistance and motivation, but be gentle.
• Monitor your breathing. Breathe slowly and rhythmically. When stretching, exhale slowly and gently stretch the muscle for about 10 to 30 seconds. Never hold your breath.
• Do not bounce. Bouncing during a stretch can increase the risk of a pulled muscle or other injury.
• Opposites attract. Always stretch opposing muscle groups such as hamstrings/quads, biceps/triceps, abs/lower back. Stretching only one of a muscle group can cause an imbalance, putting strain on one muscle and causing a decrease in flexibility.
• Try a morning stretch. Simple full-body stretches in the morning can clear your mind and help you perform more efficiently throughout the day. Taking a stretching class such as yoga or tai chi in the morning is a great way to start the day.
• Try inversion. Studies show that hanging upside down is a gentle way to stretch before or after a workout.
• Know when not to stretch. Avoid stretching without prior consent of a physician if:
• you have a recent fracture or sprain
• you have suspected or diagnosed osteoporosis
• you have inflammation around a joint
• you experience sharp, stabbing pain during stretching.

" EXPERT OPINION:

Optimal inversion is five or six minutes three times a day, moving all of your weight-bearing joints, helping them to realign themselves, re-hydrate and improve circulation generally.

— Roger Teeter, Teeter Hang Ups **"**

Chapter 7

Aging Backwards Beauty:
It's Only Epidermis Deep

It's been said that our personalities show our beauty
to the world, but looking the best we can on the
outside will only add to the overall package. As we
age, noticeable changes take place on the face and
neck and we're at the mercy of many factors, including sun, diet, genetics, lifestyle, harsh weather and our
own bad habits.

For example, smoking can produce free radicals,
once-healthy oxygen molecules that are now overac-
tive and unstable. According to Stopsmokingtoday.
com, as early as the mid-19th century it was observed
that smoking could cause visible changes in a person's
complexion, such as wrinkles, loss of elasticity and
rough or reddened complexion.

Overexposure to the sun is another way to ac-
celerate the aging process. A very high percentage of
age-associated cosmetic skin problems can be attributed to the sun. Chronic overexposure changes the
texture of the skin and weakens the elasticity. The out-
er layer of skin, or epidermis, thickens and becomes
leathery. Wrinkles, furrows, easy bruising, brown
spots, precancerous lesions and even skin cancer can
result from sun exposure. The good news is, because

photo aging of the skin is cumulative, it's never too late for a person to start a sun protection program.

I mentioned this in the chapter Aging Backwards Nutrition: Eat, Drink and Be Young, but it bears repeating. Experts believe that a lifetime of overeating sugar can cause wrinkles by damaging collagen. A high-sugar diet also affects the type of collagen you have — another factor in how resistant skin is to wrinkling. The most abundant collagen types in the skin are I, II and III, with type III being the most stable and long-lasting. Glycation, the process that occurs when you eat sugar, turns type III collagen into type I, which is more fragile, making the skin look and feel less supple. It also leaves you more vulnerable to sun damage.

Skin Pollution?

Here's an interesting factoid: Globally, dead skin accounts for about a billion tons of dust in the atmosphere. Your skin sheds 50,000 cells every minute! Anyone know where I can get a bargain gas mask?

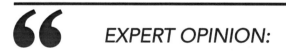 *EXPERT OPINION:*

When choosing skin care opt for quality over quantity and be consistent. Skin responds best to a simple/ consistent daily routine.

— *Francine Porter,*
Osmotics Cosmeceuticals

History Lesson

Fashion-conscious women of the second century AD in England used a moisturizer to achieve a pale and appealing look that wasn't much different from the products we use today. A few years ago, archeologists in South London unearthed a plainly decorated, sealed pot of ointment that was in good condition. In fact, finger marks left by the last person to use it were still visible on the lid. The cream was a mixture of animal fat, starch and tin oxide.

The team used the same ingredients to make a modern version of the cream, which they said goes on greasy due to the animal fat, but then turns to a smooth powdery texture, thanks to the starch. The tin oxide makes it go white when applied. Apparently the ancient "manufacturers" were health-conscious as well. Lead can be used to achieve the pale appearance, but tin oxide does it without the damaging health effects of lead.

Ageless, World's First Anti-Aging Perfume

You may have seen this in Chapter Two, Aging Backwards Fast Stats - studies show that the scent of pink grapefruit makes a man perceive a woman as younger than her age. Ageless, the world's first patent-pending anti-aging perfume from Harvey Prince & Co. in NYC, incorporates the essence of pink grapefruit with pomegranate, mango, jasmine and musk - a combination that studies prove makes men perceive women as eight years younger.

The idea behind the quest for this fragrance was simple. Company founder Kumar Ramani was inspired by the writings of Chandler Burr (perfume critic of the New York Times and author of The Perfect Scent and the Emperor of Scent). If there is a fragrance that induces one to have a migraine there had to be a fragrance that alleviated the migraine (the scent of green apple has been shown to relieve headaches). If lavender is believed to be a "calming" scent then citrus is known to be an "exciting" scent. The same is true of vanilla and peppermint. If men in focus studies and the entire fragrance industry read "rose" to be "older woman" then there has to be a fragrance that reads "younger woman." (See Chapter 14, Aging Backwards Favorites, for more information)

 EXPERT OPINION:
The Olay Definity line was created with even skin tone in mind. It actually is able to penetrate skin much deeper than most skin care products. It immediately diminishes fine lines, wrinkles and, over time, discoloration caused by hyper-pigmentation. You will see improved, even skin tone and texture.
— Bruce Grayson, makeup artist

Restylane Results

Here's some great news about the popular wrinkle filler Restylane. Research has found that not only does Restylane do a good job at filing in wrinkles, especially those pesky folds by your nose and mouth (nasolabial folds), but it also helps generate new collagen, so your skin actually repairs itself. Restylane, made in Sweden, is a clear, non-animal gel based on a natural substance called hyaluronic acid. The gel is injected into the skin in tiny amounts with a very fine needle to add volume under the wrinkles and folds to lift them up and smooth them out with immediate results and now, as we've found out, delayed results as well. It can also be used to enhance the lips.

Get The Point

Looking good is a boost to our self-esteem, but on the other hand, it may become an obsession, which can be unhealthy. So, where do we draw the line, and specifically how do we get rid of the lines?
If you're considering injections, board-certified plastic surgeon Dr. Bart Rademaker of Rejuva MedSpa in Tampa, Fla., has this advice:
• Find the right doctor. Nowadays, almost anyone will do injections. Find a board-certified physician and make sure they are using the real Botox Cosmetic brand product. Check the bottle when they remove it from the fridge.
• Don't price shop. Opting for the lowest-priced procedure could leave you with regrets. You may not be getting the amount of product you need for the best result.
• Remember your ultimate goal. The reason we get injections in the first place is to return to our natural,

youthful self, not create a new one. Do not look for a permanent solution because the rest of your face will age, but the permanently treated area will not, and you'll be left with an unsightly imbalance. Products such as Restylane and Juvederm last for six months to a year, but they will keep you looking natural.

• Know the difference. Keep in mind that Botox Cosmetic is for the "active muscle wrinkles," which are in the forehead, between the eyes and the crow's feet. Restylane and Juvederm can take care of the rest, like the nasolabial folds, those pesky parentheses by your nose, or to plump your lips.

> 66 *EXPERT OPINION:*
> *"Remember that your neck needs makeup too because makeup is part illusion using color. If makeup stops at the jaw line and the neck is a different color it destroys the illusion.*
> — *Bruce Grayson, makeup artist* 99

Beautiful Skin Tips:

• Proper face-washing habits can make a difference. Many people mistakenly think the more they wash their face, the cleaner it will be, but over-washing can strip your skin of natural oils, exacerbating the natural dryness of aging skin. Beauty experts recommend that you wash only two or three times a day at most and do not use harsh cleansers or soaps.

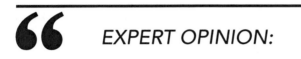 **EXPERT OPINION:**

In the islands, once a baby is born the first thing they do is cover the baby in coconut oil and every day of their lives they use coconut oil on their skin — it's a tradition.

— *Bruce Fife, C.N., N.D.*

• Stay away from cigarette smoke and that means no second-hand smoke either — and not just for your lungs.. Research has shown that exposure to cigarette smoke is as damaging to skin as exposure to the sun's ultraviolet rays. Indy Rihal of the British Skin Foundation said, "In addition to UV light from the sun and sun beds, cigarette smoke is a main environmental factor that causes changes in the skin often associated with 'looking old' such as coarse wrinkling and a sallow, leathery texture. In addition, the constriction of tiny blood vessels in the skin caused by smoking reduces the oxygen supply to the skin, negatively affecting skin health and appearance in general."

• Use a hydrating moisture cream. Contrary to popular belief, drinking water does not necessarily hydrate your skin. It's the products you use on the skin — and avoiding the harsh effects of sun, toxins in the atmosphere and smoking — that make the difference.

---

66 *EXPERT OPINION:*

Use skin care products (cosmeceuticals) based on scientifically validated technologies; these are serious products for serious results.

— Francine Porter,
Osmotics Cosmeceuticals

• Use a natural UVA/UVB sunscreen on face, neck, chest and hands. Our bodies need vitamin D and the best way to get it is from the sun. That's where my "formula" comes in. I cover my face, neck, chest and hands with sunscreen and then get a healthy glow on the rest of my body, making sure to avoid sunburn.
• Do not exfoliate too often or too harshly. Your skin can look less dull when you remove dead skin cells, but overdoing it can cause irritation, redness, dryness and flakiness.
• Choose the right makeup. As we age, we tend to want to cover up the crow's feet, deep creases and age spots that appear on our faces. Caking on makeup

is the very thing that will make any woman look older than she is. For aging skin, we should actually use a lighter touch when it comes to cosmetics. Per-fekt Skin Perfection Gel allows you to reveal your natural beauty rather than hide behind your makeup. It glides on smoothly, then turns to an airbrushed look, disguising enlarged pores, fine lines and wrinkles. You can use it alone or with your current foundation. You can even layer it to achieve just the right finish for any age.

> **EXPERT OPINION:**
> *At 40, you're dealing with issues of damage that happened earlier in your life that are now surfacing. It doesn't mean you can't cover it up with concealers, but if you start with skin care that actually works to either soften or diminish those problems, then you're working with a better canvas than you would if you didn't use anything.*
>
> — *Bruce Grayson, makeup artist*

• Use a humidifier. If you live in a dry-climate state or you use a heater during the winter, using a room humidifier can help keep your skin from drying out.

86

- Try something new. It's not necessary to keep up with every fashion trend and fad, but try not to fall into the rut of always using the same type, style and colors of makeup. For a quick and easy way to make changes, look at fashion magazines and Web sites to see what's new.
- Lose the fuzz. Unwanted facial hair growth is very common among women over age 35. Consider laser hair removal, waxing, electrolysis, shaving and/or bleaching to regain that youthful, supple, hair-free look.
- Switch from powder to cream blush. According to Bruce Grayson, Hollywood makeup artist to the stars and head of the Primetime Emmys' Makeup Department, using cream blush gives a much more natural look than powder, especially on mature skin. Bruce likes Nars' The Multiple and Clinique's Touch Blush.

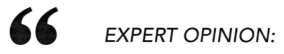 *EXPERT OPINION:*

When it comes to beautiful makeup, it's all about the condition of the skin that you're putting the makeup on. All great makeups start with beautiful skin!

— Bruce Grayson, makeup artist

All About Lasers

Are you confused about all the choices in laser cosmetic treatments available? You're not alone – there are so many different ones to treat so many different "issues," it's not easy to keep them all straight. Laser technology is being used for hair removal, skin tightening, wrinkle reduction, collagen building, cellulite reduction, age spot reduction, scars and acne, spider veins and even tattoo removal. Here's my view on lasers, which is also my view on computers: I don't have to understand how it works, I'm just happy it does. That being said, it's best to ask a trusted doctor to make recommendations for any cosmetic laser treatments you may be considering. In fact, I asked Lyda D. Tymiak, M.D. of Timeless MD Spa in Tampa Florida to explain it all and she's done just that.

Dr. Tymiak Unravels the Mystery of Lasers

Laser and light facial rejuvenation is a relatively new procedure. There were 475,000 such procedures performed in 2005 and these numbers are dramatically increasing. These cosmetic procedures can produce a clear complexion and radiant skin while minimizing lines and wrinkles. In addition, the skin is tightened and the overall look of aged skin is reduced. In 2005, there were more then 30 million light based treatments preformed. These procedures generated more then 8.5 billion dollars in gross revenues and more then seven million in equipment sales. It is predicted that by 2010 there will be more then 90 million skin rejuvenation procedures performed, increasing revenue to 15.2 billion for physicians and more than 1.1 billion in equipment sales.

The procedures are relatively quick with very little or no downtime. Bleeding and infection are uncommon as there is no incision made. Historically, skin rejuvenation started with aggressive laser treatments using the C02 laser. This caused an ablation of the full thickness of the epidermis. These lasers were popular in the mid 1990s. The trend in developing new technology has been a non-ablative type light therapy that also causes tightening of the collagen.

Lasers are instruments that produce a single wavelength of light. The wavelengths are selected depending on the tissue that is targeted. Tissues absorb certain wavelengths selectively.The wavelength selected is chosen because it is well absorbed by the target. The duration of the laser exposure is selected to allow heating of the target without damage to the surrounding tissue. Lasers are highly specific and powerful devices.

Intense Pulse Light (IPL) or broad-spectrum light is used to treat abnormal areas of the skin such as increased pigmentation, fine capillaries, actinic keratoses and acne. The broad spectrum of light can be filtered to target discreet spots, abnormal capillaries, rosacea, wrinkles and sagging skin. As skin ages, blood vessels can proliferate and become enlarged — these are termed telangiectasias. Light energy can be used to collapse these vessels without damaging surrounding skin. Vessels can be treated with intense pulse light and pulsed dye lasers. Pigmented lesions are especially well treated with lasers and light energy. Sun damage manifests as discolorations called lentigines. This color change causes a sallowness and loss of luminosity making the skin appear older. Melanin is the target in these lentigines and light energy is used to destroy the abnormal cells and pigment while leaving the normal underlying skin untouched.

Light energy only treats flat-pigmented spots. Seborrheic Keratoses or elevated lesions typically are not well treated with light and require surgical excision. Q-switched lasers such as Alexandrea Ruby and the ND Yag can also be used for precision treatment. Usually, several laser treatments are required for best results. Intense pulse light devices are used for treating discolorations of the face or body.

C02 ablative laser treatments can only be used on facial skin to the jaw line. The fractional laser applies energy in columns; however, the surrounding skin is completely left intact between the treated columns. The healthy untreated skin is the source of rapid healing.

Ablative Devices

The C02 laser is a pulse laser that is absorbed by water and vaporizes the skin. The skin must regrow over a period of seven to ten days. Significant pain is involved and there is a risk of infection. It is a treatment to re-firm deep wrinkles. Other possible complications include hypo and hyper pigmentation and scarring.

The Erbium Yag Laser is also absorbed by water. The treatment can be painful and requires topical anesthesia. The depth of treatment can vary depending on the technique. It is used for treating wrinkles and texture but does not treat pigment.

Light energy is used to treat sagging skin. ELOS Technology (Electrical Optical Synergy) uses radio frequency to preheat the skin and then infrared energy to tighten collagen. An immediate tightening effect occurs with 10% edema and 40% contraction resulting in an immediate improvement in appearance.Over a period of several weeks, collagen re-grows into the treated area and results in rejuvenated skin that is tightened with fewer wrinkles.

Radio frequency can be delivered to the skin as a point source, known as monopolar, or through two rails, known as bipolar. ELOS technology uses 3 energy sources combined into one treatment session. These energies include the SRA- RF and IPL, the Matrix Fractional Laser and the ST - Skin Tightening and Re-firming, and the RF- Bipolar Infrared.

Glossary of Terms:

Lentigines - age spots or flat tan spots caused by UV radiation also called liver spots

Freckles - flat brown spots caused by sun exposure

Malosma - facial discoloration associated with female hormones seen in pregnancy or with oral contraceptives

Seborrheic Keratoses - benign elevated skin neo-plasms: colors can range from pink to brown

Telangiectasia - irregular facial blood vessels or small bright red collections of blood usually appearing on the trunk

Leg Veins - enlarged blue veins that occur with age

Natural light - combination of visible and non-visible wavelengths

Laser light - a beam of light that is one wavelength traveling in one direction

Intense Pulse Light - broadband light that appears white but is made up of many different colors or wavelengths

ELOS Technology - Electrical Optical Synergy using technology developed by Syneron using radio frequency combined with other light energies such as intense pulse light, infrared and fractional laser

Skin SRA - ELOS technology hand piece using radio frequency and intense pulse light

Matrix - ELOS based technology using radio frequency and using fractional laser

Triniti - skin rejuvenation treatment using three hand pieces: SRA, Matrix and ST skin tightening to achieve a non-surgical face lift and skin rejuvenation

Fotofacial - patented light based treatment using ELOS and intense pulse light, Led-light emitting diode therapy, new treatment using light technology

Helpful Beauty Shortcuts
• Try facial exercises for a natural facelift. Before considering cosmetic surgery or even injections, you may want to try facial exercises to lift sagging muscles. It only makes sense to exercise the facial muscles just as you would any other muscle. Cynthia Rowland,

creator of Facial Magic and the Luscious Lips lip pump, is the expert when it comes to facial exercises and she's helped women and men look up to 15 years younger through her facial exercise program. (www.cynthiarowland.com)

• De-grease. Heat and humidity can make even the driest hair turn oily. Dawn dishwashing liquid is a well-known de-greaser. Wildlife experts even use it to save birds and marine mammals from oil spills. To get the grease out of summer hair, mix a tiny bit of Dawn detergent into your palm. Add some of your preferred shampoo. Wash, rinse and then do another wash with just the shampoo. Condition and style as usual.

 EXPERT OPINION:

In addition to its anti-bacterial, anti-viral and anti-fungal properties, coconut oil is also very cleansing and detoxifying so it will pull the toxins out of the skin.

— *Bruce Fife, C.N., N.D.*

• Unscented baby wipes make great makeup removers. Keep some in your purse or car. You might someday get caught in a rainstorm without an umbrella; no makeup looks better than rain-smeared makeup.

• Exfoliate lips by gently brushing them with a soft toothbrush, minus the toothpaste, of course.

• Wash your pillowcase every few days to keep the oils off your face. Even if you're not washing your entire bed, you can throw the pillowcase in with the towels. Choose a very soft, smooth pillowcase for the one you sleep on.

• Soften hands naturally with coconut oil. Coconut oil has been shown to be a natural disinfectant that promotes wound healing, so if you have any little cuts on your hands, you'll be treating those while you soften and moisturize.

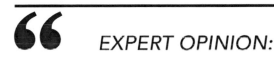

EXPERT OPINION:

In general, consumers don't have patience and are looking for a quick fix. Most of the skincare regimes that are worth the money take some time to work and see results.

— *Bruce Grayson, makeup artist*

Eye Want Beauty

"The eyes are the windows to the soul." It's an ancient proverb that dates back to biblical times and is still in use today. So, how can we make sure our "windows" always look their best?

Tips For Youthful, Beautiful Eyes

• Stop frowning. Frown lines may make you look angry, stressed, overworked or tired. Some people frown without even knowing they're doing it. I have always been very careful not to frown, so I've never developed those muscles. But if you are a frowner and you consciously pay attention, you may be able to make a habit of relaxing the space between your eyes and avoiding frowns. Some people rely on Botox Cosmetic to keep the frown lines away. Beauty expert Cynthia Rowland advocates facial exercises to keep wrinkles away.

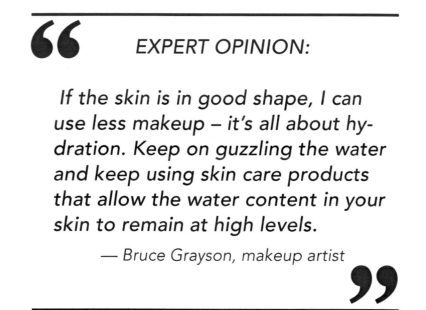

EXPERT OPINION:

If the skin is in good shape, I can use less makeup – it's all about hydration. Keep on guzzling the water and keep using skin care products that allow the water content in your skin to remain at high levels.

— *Bruce Grayson, makeup artist*

• Use concealer. Blueish under-eye circles are a result of pooled blood, while brownish or yellowish circles are the result of prior sun damage rearing its ugly head. To conceal blue circles, use a yellow shade of concealer, then apply foundation over that. For sun damage-related circles, use a peachy colored concealer.

> **" EXPERT OPINION:**
>
> *I learned this lesson from a 40-something who doesn't look a day over 19. The best way to apply eye cream (which is key to a youthful face) is with your pinky finger.*
> — Lauren Messiah, fashion expert **"**

• Lighten up. As we age, logic would tell us that we need more makeup to cover flaws. The opposite is actually true. We should wear less makeup as we get older. Bruce Grayson, Hollywood makeup artist, told me in an interview that, "less is more" when it comes to makeup for baby boomers.

• Lighten up again. Dark eye makeup colors may look nice at night, but during the day, try switching to lighter, natural shades such as peach, apricot or terra cotta, which are young and fresh looking. Avoiding glittery or shimmery shades will keep the focus off any flaws.

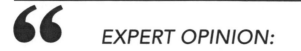 *EXPERT OPINION:*

Since eyebrows can change the look of your entire face, it's best to visit a professional for a shaping at least once every six months. Once you have the shape down you can pluck the strays hairs that pop up until your next shaping appointment.

— *Lauren Messiah, fashion expert*

• Pay attention to brows. It is perfectly acceptable to give your brows some help by adding color or length, but there are a few tips to follow to achieve the most natural result. Some experts suggest using powder shadow or eyebrow powder in a shade lighter than your hair to add color to brows, rather than using a pencil. The powder looks more natural than the "waxiness" of a pencil. Also, notice brow size.

To achieve the optimum length, hold a makeup brush from your nostril to the inner corner of the eye. Where the brush crosses the brow is where your eyebrow should start. Repeat the process, but this time, hold the brush from the nostril to the outside of the eye. This is where the brow should end.

• Go Fake. False eyelashes are back in a big way, and when done properly they can make a beautiful impact. MAC Cosmetics sells a variety of lash strips and individual lashes and they'll apply them for you for free at the time of purchase. Beauty supply stores sell strips and individual lashes that are also very affordable. They're not difficult to apply yourself if you use a magnifying mirror, tweezers and a high-quality glue formulated specifically for false eyelashes. Adding some long, fluffy lashes is a small, inexpensive way to achieve big beauty results.

EXPERT OPINION:
Way Bandy, a makeup artist that I idolized as a kid, didn't even use brushes or sponges. He used his fingers because fingers have warmth and heat up the makeup and blend it as well as a sponge.
— *Bruce Grayson, makeup artist*

The Hollywood Smile

Have you ever heard someone say, "Her smile lights up the room?" Usually they're talking about the woman to whom everyone is drawn, whether she's considered "beautiful" or not. That's because smiling can have a positive effect on everyone around you. Smiling can change your own attitude, triggering scientifically measurable activity in the left prefrontal cortex — the area of the brain where happiness and positive emotions are registered. Studies have shown that people who are smiling are perceived by others as more attractive, friendly and successful.

 EXPERT OPINION:

Teeth can show age from normal wear and tear, grinding, coffee, tea and red wine stains. Younger teeth are naturally whiter and brighter.
— *Dana Cuculici, DMD*

Good dental health is essential to a beautiful smile, but studies have shown that proper tooth and gum care is essential to heart health as well.

> **EXPERT OPINION:**
>
> *Electric toothbrushes do a much better job at removing plaque and stains than regular brushes.*
> — *Dana Cuculici, DMD*

Tips For a Healthy Mouth and Teeth

• The American Dental Association (ADA) recommends brushing your teeth twice a day with an ADA-accepted toothpaste.

> 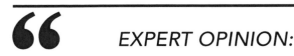 **EXPERT OPINION:**
>
> *Healthy, pink gums are a sign of a youthful smile.*
> — *Dana Cuculici, DMD*

• Replace your toothbrush every three to four months or sooner if the bristles are frayed.
• Floss daily to remove plaque and food particles from between teeth and under the gum line. Whether you brush first or floss first makes no difference, as long as you are thorough.

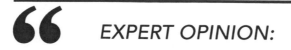

> **" EXPERT OPINION:**
>
> *Periodontal disease is an infectious disease caused by germs. Plaque and calculus are loaded with germs. The germs can get carried through the bloodstream to the heart. Periodontal disease is connected to stroke, heart attack and respiratory disease. Getting sick more often can be related to infection in the mouth.*
>
> — *Dana Cuculici, DMD* **"**

• Eat a balanced diet.
• Try tooth whiteners for discoloration, but check with your dentist for expected results because whiteners may not correct all types of discoloration. For example, yellow teeth will probably bleach well, brownish teeth may bleach less well and gray teeth will bleach even less well. Also, whiteners will not work on dental work such as bonding and white fillings.
• Be aware that certain medications, even common ones such as antihistamines, antidepressants and painkillers, can have an impact on oral health causing such side effects as dry mouth, gingivitis, soft tissue

changes and taste changes, according to the American Academy of Periodontology.

• To alleviate dry mouth, try chewing sugar-free gum and drinking more fluids.

• Sugary lollipops have long been associated with tooth decay, but a new lollipop has been developed to kill the bacteria that cause tooth decay. Marketed as Dr. John's Herbal Candy, the orange-flavored, sugar-free lollipops are actually good for your teeth.

They're infused with a natural ingredient found in licorice that kills the bacteria that are the primary cause of tooth decay, Streptococcus mutans. The same concept is also being applied to targeting bacteria in the nose, ear and gut, to name a few. Sweet!

" EXPERT OPINION:

The idea that the smile can enhance beauty goes back to ancient times. Ancient Babylonians decorated their teeth by encrusting them with diamonds and rubies.

— *Dana Cuculici, DMD*

Hair Today

We spend countless hours — not to mention dollars — trying to improve the appearance of aging skin, but what about our hair? As we age, our hair loses its color and can appear dull, faded and coarse. Factors that can age hair include sun and harsh weather, hormonal changes, chemical treatments, heat styling, lack of protein and the natural slow-down of cell regeneration. Even certain medications such as high blood pressure and cholesterol medicines can age hair.

 EXPERT OPINION:

For women over 50 who want long hair, it's not so much the length of the hair, it's the color and the cut. I think longer cuts can work for older women. I wouldn't have a woman over 50 wearing bangs, but if you do wear bangs, you want them to blend into the hairstyle.

-- Bruce Grayson, makeup artist

Aging Backwards Happy Hair Tips
• Choose the right hairstyle. Having a hairstyle that flatters your face and shows your personality is one way to look younger. Look through magazines for hairstyles and pick out styles you like on people who have hair similar to yours, regardless of their ages. Bring them to a hairstylist you trust and let them guide you and give you the best cut for your face shape and hair type.

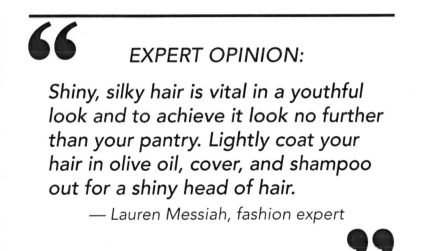

66 *EXPERT OPINION:*

Shiny, silky hair is vital in a youthful look and to achieve it look no further than your pantry. Lightly coat your hair in olive oil, cover, and shampoo out for a shiny head of hair.
— *Lauren Messiah, fashion expert*
99

• Check your iron levels. Non-genetic hair loss is much worse in women who are deficient in iron and those who have low levels of B vitamins. Nine out of 10 women aged 16 to 50 and one in three women over 50 are deficient in iron.

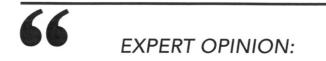

> ## EXPERT OPINION:
>
> *Of the 70 million people who are suffering from hair loss, approximately 40 million are women. That is an epidemic proportion.*
> — *Jacqueline Tarrant, hair expert*

• Go natural. If you constantly use heat to dry and style your hair, trying letting it dry naturally whenever possible. When it's almost dry, you can roll it up in large Velcro rollers to smooth and style without heat or damage.

• Rinse with cold. For shiny hair, give it a final rinse with cold water. This will close the cuticle and leave a smooth, shiny surface. Using the cold-blast button on the blow dryer has a similar smoothing effect.

• Go easy on products. Less is more when it comes to hair products and that includes shampooing. Washing hair every day can strip it of natural oils. If possible, try shampooing every other day and use light, alcohol-free products that won't weigh down your hair.

> **"**   *EXPERT OPINION:*
>
> *There is nothing natural about hair dye, we all know that, but covering up grays with hair color that screams, 'I came from a box' is a no-no. Choose a natural color dye and people won't know the difference. A 60-year-old woman with dyed cherry red hair is better off gray, trust me.*
>
> — Lauren Messiah, fashion expert   **"**

• Try a different style. Thanks to the digital age, you can "try on" hairstyles by uploading your photo to virtual try-on studios. Just type "virtual hairstyles" into Google and you'll get about 195,000 results. Take your pick.

• Try a different color. Clairol.com has a color quiz that will help you match your color to your "inner beauty."

• Go wig shopping. Want to change your hairstyle temporarily for special occasions? Keep some cute wigs in your closet and transform your look whenever you want for as long as you want.

EXPERT OPINION:

Women are masters of disguise, so as a result, many times women are quietly suffering with hair loss and people are unaware.

— Jacqueline Tarrant, hair expert

• Try scalp massage. Massaging the scalp enhances blood circulation and helps strengthen the roots of the hair, promoting new hair growth. Not only does the massage work wonders for your hair, but it also relaxes the mind and nervous system.

• Nourish your hair. Eating a well-balanced diet is not just good for your body — it's good for your hair, too. One particularly hair friendly food is seaweed. Some people even claim it helps to re-grow hair. According to research, seaweed promotes the growth of thicker, more lustrous hair.

So, if you're feeling adventuresome, try something different with your hair and remember — it's only hair. If you experiment and hate the style, it grows back. If you experiment with the color and change your mind, just re-color it. Hair is one of the few things we can afford to make mistakes with and not regret, at least not permanently.

> *EXPERT OPINION:*
> *Traction alopecia is the fastest growing category in the hair loss platform and that's something we can avoid. When we pull ponytails back and wear them too tight or when women wear braided styles or hair extensions, the trauma that is experienced down in the hair root from that tension causes hair loss.*
> — *Jacqueline Tarrant, hair expert*

Dos and Don'ts For Dressing Young

The first rule of dressing young is to avoid looking as if you're "trying" to look trendy. The trick to looking "in the season," is to buy one or two pieces from the newest look and mix them in with your classic wardrobe. Every season has its latest hot look, whether it's a certain color, skirt length, purse or shoe. Keep in mind price when purchasing the trendy pieces, since they'll likely go out of fashion just as quickly as they came in.

The talent for mixing and matching wardrobe pieces is not something everyone is born with and some people simply don't have time for "power shopping." That's where this shortcut comes into play: take advantage of personal shoppers at stores such as Nordstrom or others in your area. Not only will they save you precious time, but they're trained to really help you make smart wardrobe choices. If you can't find a store near you that offers personal shoppers, take along a friend who has an artistic eye and whom you trust to tell you the truth about which looks are flattering and which ones should go back on the rack.

Another trick to dressing younger is to update the styles of some of your wardrobe staples. For example, if black pants are your favorite, swap out your usual black pants for a new pair that has the look of the season, whether it's a cuff, pleat or new waistline. You can still pair the black pants with your favorite tops, but now you've created a slightly trendier look.

Add some inexpensive but classy accessories of the season, a cute bag and the latest shoes, and you're fitting right in with the younger women. I always say, "Don't spend a fortune on designer clothes." Most younger women can't afford those exclusive pieces. Watch the way younger women dress and make an effort to emulate them in a subtle way. Refer back to the number one rule: you don't want to look as if you're trying too hard.

Finally, for a quick and easy way to stay current, go online to Marie Claire or Glamour Web sites or pick up a fashion magazine once a month, or at least once a season, to see the latest looks.

Oui Love French Manicures

A French manicure is a classic, clean look that never goes out of style. It is the preferred manicure for brides because it's very feminine and glamorous. The French manicure has been called, "The ultimate in sophistication," by style experts. The origin of the French manicure is difficult to trace, but manicures themselves have been around for more than 4,000 years. The use of fingernail polish can be traced back to China in 3000 BC, when nail color indicated one's social status.

A citation in a Ming Dynasty manuscript pointed out that royal fingernails were painted black and red. The Egyptians also used red nails to denote the highest social class. Some historians claim that famous makeup artist Max Factor invented the French manicure for the fashionable ladies of Paris in the 1930s. What is known is that the Los Angeles-based company Orly trademarked the term "Original French Manicure" in 1978.

Help For Hands

After the face, hands are the second most visible telltale sign of one's age, according to the American Society of Plastic Surgeons. There are laser treatments for age spots and injections for thin, spidery hands. But here's an Aging Backwards tip for instantly younger hands that's affordable, quick and easy: Studies show that nail polish and jewelry make hands appear younger. Volunteers were shown photos of hands without jewelry and without polish and photos of the same hands with jewelry and polish. The majority thought the hands looked younger with polish and jewelry. So, get a manicure and wear a ring, and voila — instantly younger hands.

The Vein of My Existence

Nearly 20 percent of all adult women and 10 percent of all adult men are affected by varicose veins, to some degree. For many people they are a family trait. Although they can appear anywhere, they usually affect the legs and feet. Varicose veins can often be painful, perhaps unsightly, can become tender to the touch and can hinder circulation when inflamed. This causes a myriad of symptoms including aching legs and feet, itchiness, swollen ankles and even discolored, peeling skin.

Varicose veins are caused by a variety of conditions, including dietary deficiency, heavy lifting, hormonal changes due to pregnancy or aging, having a job that requires prolonged sitting or standing, lack of exercise, obesity, genetics, and even tight clothing. Good news, though — your doctor can get rid of them. Many doctors are now using lasers to remove spider veins and sclerotherapy to treat superficial varicose veins. For the latter, a sclerosing agent (chemical) is injected into the vein to collapse its walls so it can no longer transport blood. In severe cases, the vein may be surgically removed, but no treatment can prevent new veins from becoming varicose.

High Heel Heaven

Here's some news for shoe divas: Wearing 2-inch heels puts your foot at a 15-degree angle to the ground, which also happens to put your pelvis into the perfect position to improve the strength of those Kegel muscles that are so important to supporting the bladder, bowels and uterus. The same muscles are associated with a satisfying sexual experience. These muscles often weaken after pregnancy and childbirth, and as we age. These findings shouldn't be taken as a license to stop doing Kegel exercises, but it's good to know wearing heels may have the potential health benefit of strengthening the pelvic floor muscles.

Chapter 8

The Aging Backwards Brain:
It's All in Your Head

Think thin, be thin. Many studies have been done that prove your thoughts do influence your life. Try a new way of thinking if you've got some pounds to shed. Instead of thinking: "I've got to lose 10 pounds to fit into that dress," change your thinking to: "I want to lose 10 pounds for myself to look better and feel better." Instead of: "I'll just have a couple of cookies," try: "Why tempt myself with cookies? I know it's hard to stop, so I won't even have one." Instead of: "Ugh, time to work out again, I just hate this," why not think: "I'm going to have a great workout and feel energized and fantastic when it's over."

Numbers Game

Today's technology is making us dumber. According to a survey conducted by researchers from Puzzler Brain Trainer magazine and reported by Reuters, all those cell phones and portable devices that store gobs of personal information have created a generation incapable of memorizing simple things. A quarter of those polled said they couldn't remember their landline number, while two-thirds couldn't recall the birthdays of more than three friends or family members.

In case you're wondering, this isn't because of aging. In fact, the tech-savvy under-30s could remember fewer birthdays and numbers than the over-50s.

Use It or Lose It

We've all heard that phrase about a million times, but when it comes to your brain, it's good advice. Many studies have been done on the "aging brain," including one called the MacArthur Study of Successful Aging that identified 1,200 healthy people between the ages of 70 and 80 whose mental abilities ranked in the top third compared to others in the same age group. They kept track of these participants for 10 years and determined which people remained high functioning. The results showed three factors separated the high functioning subjects from the others:

• They were more consistently physically active, taking daily walks or doing other types of exercise.
• They remained mentally active, doing crossword puzzles, reading interesting books, playing bridge three times a week and engaging in hobbies.
• They met challenges with confidence, rather than buckling under misfortune.

Social Studies

Socializing is good for your brain. According to a recent study, spending just 10 minutes talking to another person can improve your memory as well as your performance on tests. Researchers from the University of Michigan found that the higher the level of social interaction of the study volunteers, the better their cognitive functioning, no matter what their age. The study participants ranged in age from 24 to 96. "In our study, socializing was just as effective as more traditional kinds of mental exercise in boosting memory and intellectual performance," said Oscar Ybarra, a psychologist at the University of Michigan Institute for Social Research and a lead author of the study, along with colleague Eugene Burnstein and psychologist Piotr Winkelman from the University of California at San Diego.

EXPERT OPINION:

In older people who have decreased circulation to the brain, inversion can help bring the circulation of the brain up to where it should be.
— *Roger Teeter, Teeter Hang Ups*

Brain Workout

Just as your muscles benefit from exercise, so does your brain — studies have proven it time and again. One such study involved 23 healthy people, average age 23, who were taught to juggle. After three months, MRI scans showed enlargement of the gray matter in their brains. Gray matter is responsible for higher mental functioning. When the participants stopped juggling, their brains shrank again, strongly suggesting that mental exercise has valid positive effects on brain function.

It's Who You Know
Crossword puzzles are a terrific way to sharpen your brain and besides, they're fun. If you've never enjoyed crossword puzzles, it could be because you don't know the "insider secret." On Monday, the puzzle is the easiest and it gets progressively more difficult later in the week. This is true for virtually every newspaper. So if you're a crossword novice, try the Monday puzzle first.

Many people have free time on the weekend, so they pick up the Saturday or Sunday puzzle and find it impossible. Start with baby steps on Monday. Also, if you can't finish the puzzle, put it down and pick it up again the following day. You'll be surprised at how easily the tough answers from yesterday can come to you. My crossword "guru" and good friend is Merl Reagle. He's even created the original Aging Backwards crossword puzzle on the next page.

Aging Backwards
Crossword Puzzle
By Merl Reagle
(answers on page 170)

119

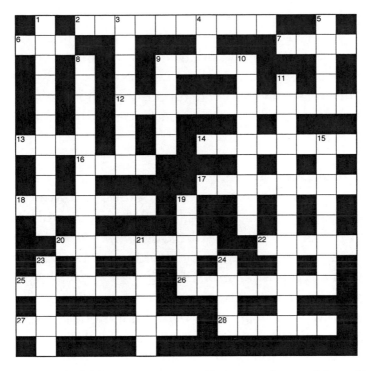

ACROSS

2 Nature's tropical skin softener
6 Good way to enjoy your 25 Across
7 Battle of the bulge?
9 Vegetarian's protein source
12 Pomegranates and blueberries pack them in
13 ___ a health club
14 Iron these out!
16 Weightlifting will do this to your body
17 The best medicine
18 People who are there for you
20 A, B, C, D, & E
22 More than just "not good for you"
25 Nutrient-rich natural foods, for short
26 Night creams and more

27 It gets to the root of the problem
28 It comes in pretty colors

DOWN

1 Those born 1946 to 1964
3 It gets under your skin
4 It's red, white, green, or black
5 Your body's pump
8 Helping others that's good for your soul
9 It'll take the frown off your face
10 Your "keeping the faith" side
11 It's more beneficial than the milk ilk
15 Run, jump, step, spin, crunch
19 Air bags?
21 Quadriceps, for one
23 Grounds for a good night's sleep?
24 Like a youthful body

Don't Stress Your Memory

When high levels of the stress hormone cortisol are released into the bloodstream, you can experience memory loss and confusion, according to a study done at Saint Louis University. Fortunately, as the levels of cortisol decreased, the study participants' memories improved.

Train-Your-Brain Tricks

• Say it aloud. Try this tip for remembering where you place your keys, phone, etc. When you set down your phone, tell yourself out loud where it is. "My cell phone is in the kitchen." Try it with your keys and any other item you usually misplace.

• Memorize outdoor boards and signs. I like to train my brain while I'm stuck in traffic. I'll memorize phone numbers and other information I see on billboards, just to exercise my gray matter.

• If you're right-handed, try a left-handed day, and vice versa if you're left-handed. It will feel awkward at first, but after a while you'll get accustomed to the switch and you'll find that being ambidextrous can come in handy, especially if your dominant hand is ever out of commission due to a cast or a nasty cut.

• Exercise. Investigators from the Howard Hughes Medical Institute (HHMI) have found that exercise improves learning and memory. "Until recently it was thought that the growth of new neurons, or neuro-genesis, did not occur in the adult mammalian brain," said Terrence Sejnowski, an HHMI investigator at the Salk Institute for Biological Studies. "But we now have evidence for it, and it appears that exercise helps this happen."

• Use acrostics. An acrostic can be a very simple way to remember a list of words, such as your grocery list. For example, if you need to buy milk, fruit, veggies, eggs and nuts, your sentence could be: "My First Very Excellent Name," using the first letter of each word to create the sentence.

• Use association. This is especially helpful in remembering names. If, for example, you are introduced to someone named Ryan Fields you could use the association, "Eat rye bread in the field."

• Sing a song. Most of us don't even bother to learn phone numbers anymore. We simply store the number in our cell phone or PDA, search our contact list and press "send." However, if you find yourself without your mobile device, you may want to have certain numbers in your head. This happened to me in New York City.

    I left my phone at the apartment of the friend I was staying with then I ventured out on my own. She was to meet me later, but I realized that in case of emergency, I didn't even know her phone number! I had called her hundreds of times, but never bothered to learn the number. Putting the numbers to the tune of a song can help. "Three Blind Mice" is a nice choice for phone numbers because it's 10 syllables and phone numbers contain 10 numbers (area code included). So, you could match the numbers to the tune of: "Three blind mice, three blind mice, see how they run." And … remember not to forget what you were trying to remember by using these tips!

EXPERT OPINION:

As people age, they start limiting their activities, so they need to set goals. They start saying to themselves, 'I'm too old,' 'I can't do this,' 'I haven't got time to finish that,' 'It takes too much energy,' and they need to get rid of that stinkin' thinkin'.

— *Roger Y. Murray, M.D.*

Chapter 9
Aging Backwards Overnight:
Sleep Secrets

atch your Zzzs. Count sheep. Get your beauty rest. Crash out. Sleep tight. Whichever way you say it, getting your beauty sleep is conducive to Aging Backwards.

 EXPERT OPINION:

A single night of reduced sleep significantly impairs your ability to function. As you add days, impairment becomes cumulative. Even more alarming is lack of sleep contributes to diabetes, obesity, weakened immune system, depression, cancer, high blood pressure, heart disease and stroke.

— *David A. Kekich,*
Maximum Life Foundation

Sleep Yourself Smart

My friends always marvel at the way I remember all the names of their men and relatives and how I keep straight all the details of their dramas. Now I know why — I sleep eight hours a night. A study revealed that getting your beauty rest could have more benefits than just beauty. Researchers found that getting enough sleep may also sharpen your memory. In the study, the researchers focused on sleep's impact on "declarative memories," which deal with specific facts, episodes and events — hence my remembering all the details of my friends' dramas.

"We sought to explore whether sleep has any impact on memory consolidation, specifically the type of memory for facts and events and time," explained Dr. Jeffrey Ellenbogen, an associate neurologist at Brigham and Women's Hospital in Boston and a post-doctoral fellow in sleep medicine at Harvard Medical School. "We know that sleep helps boost memory for procedural tests, such as learning a new piano sequence, but we're not sure, even though it's been debated for 100 years, whether sleep impacts declarative memory." Now we know ... it does. Nighty night!

Sleep Yourself Thin

A recent study found there's a specific range of sleep that can keep you thin. It's a Canadian study from Laval University in Quebec, which revealed that too little sleep could lead to weight gain — and too much sleep can also lead to weight gain. According to the study, seven to eight hours of sleep is the magic number — no more, no less. In the study, people who slept five or six hours a night were 35 percent more likely to gain 11 pounds over a six-year period and people who slept nine or 10 hours a night were 25 percent more likely to gain 11 pounds over the same period than the ones who slept seven to eight hours.

 EXPERT OPINION:

It's extremely easy to measure hormonal levels, nutrition and toxicities. Instead of guessing, the best thing to do is to measure.

— *Sangeeta Pati, M.D.*

Man vs. Woman

A study found that women sleep less soundly when they share a bed with a romantic partner while men actually sleep better when they snuggle up next to a woman. A man's snoring is one obvious detriment to a woman's beauty rest, but it's not the only one. According to researchers, women tend to be lighter sleepers in general, perhaps because they are the ones, historically, who take care of infants.

Psychologist Wendy Troxel, a researcher at the University of Pittsburgh, explained that another reason why men sleep better with a woman beside them is because studies show that men are very dependent on close relationships. Statistics show that married men are much happier and healthier than single men. The same can't always be said for women, though, according to the studies.

Aging Backwards Tips for Sleep
• Keep your room dark. Get heavy curtains that block out light or wear a soft sleep mask.
• Use sound. Studies show that ambient sound, such as a fan or air conditioner, can lull you to sleep. In fact, there are machines you can buy that provide numerous sounds, from ocean waves to white noise and even the sound of a heart beating for infants.
• Wear earplugs. Unlike ambient, soothing sounds, nighttime noise, such as planes flying overhead, can raise your blood pressure even while you're asleep, according to a study out of Europe. High blood pressure has been associated with increased risk of heart disease, kidney disease, stroke and even dementia. The researchers studied 140 volunteers who were monitored at home while they slept. Sounds such as airplane noise, traffic noise or a partner snoring raised the participants' blood pressure even while they were asleep and totally unaware of the noise.

Dr. Lars Jarup, one of the authors of the study from the Department of Epidemiology and Public Health at Imperial College London, said, "We know that noise from air traffic can be a source of irritation, but our research shows that it can also be damaging for people's health, which is particularly significant in light of plans to expand international airports. Our studies show that nighttime aircraft noise can affect your blood pressure instantly and increase the risk of hypertension. It is clear to me that measures need to be taken to reduce noise levels from aircraft, in particular during nighttime, in order to protect the health of people living near airports."

• Wash your pillowcases often. Washing your pillowcases often will soften them so they won't be as wrinkle producing. Also, the oils from your face transfer to
your pillowcase. I throw mine in with the towels, which
get washed more often than the sheets.
• Try melatonin. The body's level of the hormone melatonin normally increases after darkness falls, making
you feel drowsy. If you suffer from insomnia, metalonin
may help you fall asleep and stay asleep. Melatonin has
numerous other benefits, such as boosting the immune
system and protecting from free radical damage with
its antioxidant content. It's also used as a treatment for
jet lag. So, if you have trouble sleeping occasionally, try
one or more of these tips. If you have chronic trouble
sleeping, consult your doctor or get help from the National Sleep Foundation, (202) 347-3471.

Chapter 10
Aging Backwards Stress Relief:
Finding Tranquility

 EXPERT OPINION:

Exercise on a regular basis and use mind-body interactions to reduce psychological stress.

— *Stephen T. Sinatra, M.D.*

Some people are natural worriers and I confess I'm one of those. In my younger years, I'd worry about what other people were thinking of me — what I wore, what I said, what I didn't say. I think I even worried that I wasn't worrying enough! I could always put on a confident facade so most people around me never knew the extent of my "affliction." You become an expert at hiding things after a while.

Then one day I was visiting a friend and discovered a beautiful framed poster on her bathroom wall. If you didn't look at it closely, it seemed like just a jumble of sentences all running together, handwritten in an artsy fashion, but buried in the middle was a gem. It read: "90 percent of everything I worry about never happens." Wow, I found that to be so true! I took that sentence and made it my own personal mantra. I still worry sometimes, even about totally insignificant things, but then I repeat my mantra: "90 percent of everything I worry about never happens," and the worries dissipate.

Another great way for coping with worry and stress that I've discovered is through Emotional Freedom Techniques (EFT), founded by Gary Craig. This method, which has been recommended by medical doctors, is based on the concepts of acupuncture and acupressure by focusing on the energy meridian points of the body. EFT uses a series of tapping and "statements" that many people have used to relieve pain, improve performance in sports and unblock emotional issues, to name a few. It's simple to learn – even children are using it. You can find out more about EFT and download a free guide at www.emofree.com.

EXPERT OPINION:

If we're under a lot of stress, many of our hormones can become out of balance earlier. It's how we react to and handle internal and external stresses. We need to reduce the plague of the 21st century — stress.

— Sangeeta Pati, M.D.

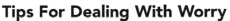

Tips For Dealing With Worry
• Focus on your senses. Stroke your pet's soft fur, listen to soothing music, breathe in the scent of flowers or freshly-baked cinnamon buns, watch kids play. Focusing on pure sensations can help take your mind off of what's troubling you.
• Keep a gratitude journal. Writing down the things you're thankful for can have great benefits. Research studies show that people who kept gratitude journals felt better about the upcoming week than those who kept track of hassles or even neutral events.
• Fake a smile. A study from Clark University in Worcester, Mass., revealed that students who made frowning expressions by pushing their eyebrows together felt angry, even when watching cartoons, but those who were induced to smile felt happier and found the cartoons funnier.

• Sniff peppermint. According to Dr. Alan Hirsch, founder and neurological director of the Smell & Taste Treatment and Research Foundation in Chicago, breathing in the scent of peppermint will make you "more awake and alert, and that leads to feeling upbeat."

• Look through your photo albums. Immersing yourself in a trip down memory lane can take your mind off of current worries, reminding you of all you've experienced and achieved.

• Don't wait for someone to bring you flowers. Enjoy them anytime by buying them or picking them from your own garden.

• Practice yoga, qi gong, tai chi, meditation, visualization and/or relaxation techniques.

 EXPERT OPINION:

Our brains are too big for our own good health — we push ourselves too much, we ruminate, we worry and we have a society that's built on stimulation. Too much change, too high of a pace, it's all interpreted as stress by our bodies. We need to reverse those stresses for aging backwards.

— *Al Sears, M.D.*

Stress Ages You

It's been proven that chronic stress can cause premature aging. Elissa Epel, Ph.D., and her colleagues from the University of California, San Francisco's Psychiatry Department, found that while hormonal changes are a normal part of aging, chronic stress could affect hormone levels and alter the body's delicate hormonal balance. You're probably familiar with some stress relieving techniques such as yoga and deep breathing, but why not try something different? When we're stressed, we tend to clench our teeth, causing pain and stiffness in the jaw that can lead to headaches, neck pain, even back pain. Try massaging the jaw muscle underneath your ears for relief.

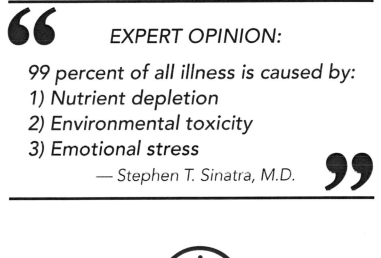

EXPERT OPINION:

99 percent of all illness is caused by:
1) Nutrient depletion
2) Environmental toxicity
3) Emotional stress
— Stephen T. Sinatra, M.D.

Chapter 11

Aging Backwards Longevity:
Optimal Octogenarian Years

The popular quote "Life Begins at 40" was actually the title of a 1933 best-selling book by author W.B. Pitkin. These days, you could probably say life begins at 70, 80 or even 90.

❝ **EXPERT OPINION:**

Anti-aging medicine is trying to extend the youthful, productive life span of everyone.

— *Ronald Klatz, M.D.*

Ya Gotta Have Friends

A study reported in the British Medical Journal found that friends could be a more important factor in helping seniors live longer. About 1,500 participants were asked about their social networks including how much personal and phone contact they had with their friends, children and other relatives. Then their survival rates were tracked for 10 years. Close ties with children and other family members apparently had no impact on longevity, but those who had a very strong personal network of close friends and confidants showed much higher survival rates.

The reason? Family ties can often be maintained out of a sense of obligation, while friendships are a matter of choice. The researchers also found that children often have little influence over habits such as smoking and drinking, but the opinions of friends and peers weigh much higher in importance.

 EXPERT OPINION:

When your cells are working properly, there's little in the way of disease that creeps up on you.
— *Ronald Klatz, M.D.*

It's Never Too Late to Start Aging Backwards

Even those who begin adopting a healthy lifestyle in middle age can lower their risk of heart disease by 35 percent and lower their risk of premature death by 40 percent within four years of changing their lifestyle, according to a study led by Dr. Dana King at the Medical University of South Carolina. The study found that middle-aged adults who added five fruits and vegetables a day to their diets, began exercising at least 2-1/2 hours a week, maintained a healthy weight and didn't smoke achieved those phenomenal results. "The adopters of a healthy lifestyle basically caught up. Within four years, their mortality rate and rate of heart attacks matched the people who had been doing these behaviors all along," said Dr. King.

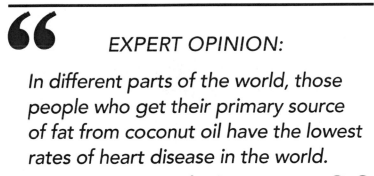

EXPERT OPINION:

In different parts of the world, those people who get their primary source of fat from coconut oil have the lowest rates of heart disease in the world.

— *Bruce Fife, C.N., N.D.*

Stretching: The Key to Longevity?

Using inversion, or hanging upside down, is a gentle way to stretch, but it also has numerous additional health benefits. Studies show that inversion can decompress your spine and help you maintain your height. According to Roger Teeter, founder and president of Teeter Hang Ups, most people will lose from a half inch to 2 inches in height during their lifetime due to thinning discs. As a baby, your discs are 90 percent water. However, the water content in the discs decreases to 70 percent by age 70. An active inversion program could help maintain more of your original height.

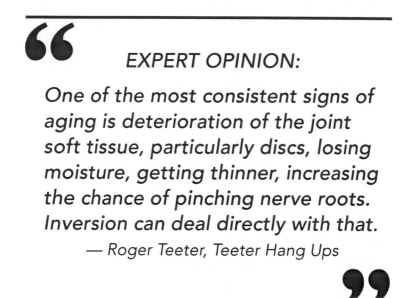

> **" EXPERT OPINION:**
>
> *One of the most consistent signs of aging is deterioration of the joint soft tissue, particularly discs, losing moisture, getting thinner, increasing the chance of pinching nerve roots. Inversion can deal directly with that.*
> — *Roger Teeter, Teeter Hang Ups* **"**

Other health benefits to be gained by using the inversion table include increased oxygen to the brain, decongestion of internal organs, relief of varicose veins, improved posture, stress relief, reduction in back pain, strengthening of ligaments, and the list goes on. Plus, it just plain feels good! People with certain health conditions should not invert, so always check with your doctor first.

EXPERT OPINION:

It's normal for most 100-year-olds to be in a box in the ground. Does that mean you want to be 'normal?' Well, I don't. So, we came up with anti-aging medicine because that's exactly what we're trying to do — we're trying to defy aging and defy the degeneration that occurs with aging.

— *Ronald Klatz, M.D.*

Contagious — in a Good Way

Harvard researchers have found that quitting smoking is contagious. According to the research, a smoker is more likely to quit if a spouse, friend, sibling or co-worker kicks the habit. When a spouse stops smoking, the other partner is 67 percent less likely to smoke. When a friend quits, the odds of the other continuing drops by 36 percent. The odds are similar among co-workers and siblings. Smoking still contributes to the deaths of 435,000 Americans a year and, according to the Centers for Disease Control and Prevention (CDC), 50,000 of those deaths can be attributed to secondhand smoke.

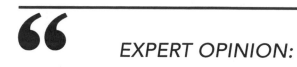

EXPERT OPINION:

If you are invested in mutual funds, retirement funds, hedge funds, the chances are, you are invested in what I sometimes call 'pro-death industries.' They include fast foods, processed foods, alcoholic and soft drinks, and tobacco.

— David A. Kekich,
Maximum Life Foundation

Free To Be Me

I just thought I'd remind you that there are plenty of things you can do to start Aging Backwards that are so affordable, you can do them every day — they're free! That's why they're in the longevity chapter. You can do them forever and they won't cost you an arm and a leg; in fact, they'll benefit your arms, legs and more!

• Exercise. By now you're probably getting tired of hearing me tout exercise, exercise, exercise, but studies continue to show that regular exercise keeps you young and healthy. Instead of telling you to exercise, I'm going to offer some ways to motivate you.

I love to work out, but even I want to be a couch

potato sometimes. When the couch potato syndrome comes over me, I "fake" the workout. By that I mean that I tell myself I'm just going to "play along," go through the motions and not really work out, but at least I won't be sitting around. So, I don the cutest outfit I can find in my closet, put on my sneaks and set out to exercise, whether it's a brisk walk, one of my favorite workout DVDs or going to the gym. (The walk is free.) No matter how tired or lethargic I feel, five minutes into the workout I find new energy and get into the groove. Try it.

Here's another trick I use to motivate myself: I'll go online and look at beautiful clothes or workout sites where people with beautifully healthy bodies are exercising and that reminds me that in order to keep Aging Backwards, I have to get moving. If they can do it, so can I.

• Sleep. Another subject I talk about constantly is beauty rest, but that's because it's so important. Sleep is free — take advantage of that. When we sleep, our bodies produce hormones that keep us healthy and youthful. Why pay for hormones when you can get them for free?

• Water. Recent studies have debunked the 8x8 (eight, eight-ounce glasses) water myth, but I don't think anyone can argue that pure, fresh water is good for us. According to a recent report, drinking eight glasses of water a day does not necessarily improve skin tone nor is it required for good health.

Still, I'm Aging Backwards and I love to drink my pure, fresh water (free from the tap and not all tap water is "bad," plus it keeps those plastic bottles out of the eco-system). It is possible to drink too much water — people have even died from water intoxication (hyponatremia) so pacing yourself and listening to your body is the best advice.

• Laughter. Can laughing keep you Aging Backwards and fight heart disease? According to researchers at the University of Maryland School of Medicine it can. A study done by cardiologists at the school revealed, "People with heart disease responded less humorously to everyday life situations," according to lead researcher Dr. Michael Miller. He added, "The recommendation for a healthy heart may one day be exercise, eat right and laugh a few times a day."

EXPERT OPINION:
The thing you notice about older people is they become negative and grumpy, they lose their social graces. One of the important aspects of anti-aging is you have to give yourself — and your mate — positive affirmations and stay in the positive.
— Roger Murray, M.D.

• Meditation. "Mindfulness meditation programs improve mood and health," said David Creswell, a UCLA psychologist and lead researcher in a study published in Psychosomatic Medicine. When Creswell and his team compared the brains of people who had mindful dispositions with those who were considered less mindful, there were measurable differences in their brain activity. The mindful subjects' brains showed more activity in the right prefrontal cortex and a calming of the amygdala (the region responsible for emotional processing) when they labeled their emotions.

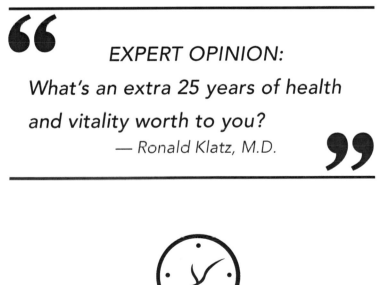

EXPERT OPINION:

What's an extra 25 years of health

and vitality worth to you?
— *Ronald Klatz, M.D.*

Chapter 12
Aging Backwards Spirit:
The Renewed Soul

EXPERT OPINION:
"As we get older, we stop doing things that make us feel good. One thing I like to do is pay the toll for the person behind me."
— *Roger Y. Murray, M.D.*

Numerous scientific studies show that acts of kindness can result in significant mental and physical health benefits. Helping can bring on a rush of euphoria, followed by a longer period of calm, often called a "helper's high" that releases the body's natural painkiller, endorphins, thus reversing feelings of depression, hostility and stress. Reducing stress can have such health benefits as reducing obesity, sleeplessness, acid stomach, backache, headache and more, according to the Random Acts of Kindness Foundation.

Volunteerism Happy Stats
• The greater the frequency of volunteering, the greater the health benefits.
• Personal contact with the people being helped is important.
• Helper's high results most from helping people we don't know.
• Regular club attendance, volunteering, entertaining or faith group attendance is the happiness equivalent of getting a college degree or more than doubling your income.

A Century of Good Health
       A survey of people over 100 years old reveals that faith and spirituality were cited most often as the source of their longevity, according to a survey sponsored by a unit of UnitedHealth Group. In a survey of 100 people between the ages of 100 and 104, 23 percent said faith, rather than genes and good medical care, were responsible for their long life. Hard work, a healthy diet and "living a good, clean life" were other factors also mentioned.
       Sixty-one percent of those surveyed said there was nothing they would have done more of in their lives and 78 percent said there was nothing they would have done less. About 13 percent said they wished they had traveled more; 9 percent said they wished they had worked less; and 6 percent said they wished they had spent more time with their families. The survey also revealed that 30 percent of centenarians considered raising a family as their most satisfying achievement while 20 percent put the most value on their careers.

EXPERT OPINION:

How old are you now? Uh, uh. Not so fast. If your first impulse was to tell me how many years it has been since you were born, stop right there. There could be a huge difference between your chrono- logical age and your biological age. And you have control over that difference.

— *David A. Kekich,*
Maximum Life Foundation

Dolphin Therapists

Swimming is an excellent form of exercise, but did you know swimming with dolphins is good for your soul? There's actually been a study done and research- ers found that an hour a day in the water with those sociable creatures is an effective treatment for mild to moderate depression — even better than swimming with other humans! Psychiatrists from the University of Leicester compared two groups of patients suffering from depression.

Half of the group swam and snorkeled with dolphins while the other half spent the same amount of time swimming and snorkeling with each other but without dolphins. Participants in the study stopped taking any kind of antidepressants four weeks before the study and their levels of depression were measured. After two weeks, results showed that the group who swam with the dolphins had a much more significant improvement than the group who swam without Flipper.

Not only that, but after three months, the group who swam with dolphins reported lasting improvement in their depression symptoms and no longer needed treatment.

Uplifting Tips
Here are some tips to keep you going when it feels as if nothing is right.
• Try to think of something you can feel grateful about, whether it's good health, your children or a loving relationship.
• Take time out to do some exercise, even if it's only for 10 minutes. Remember, this is exercise to help your mind at the moment, so even 10 minutes can make a big difference.
• Change the subject. When you're fuming about something, immerse yourself in a separate, unrelated activity. You'd be surprised at how easily you can calm down.
• If you have a pet, seek him out for a play session or a luxurious brushing. Animals have a calming effect on people.

• Check out the comics section in your local news-paper or go online and find a joke Web site. A good laugh can be very healing.

• Go online to CharityNavigator.com to see all the ways you can give back. Helping those less fortunate is a feel-good activity.

• Write down your good qualities and re-read the list. It will remind you that there are many positives in your life.

• Discover Voluntourism. That's no typo — it's the newest trend in vacationing. More and more people are opting to "give back" on their vacation time, choosing trips with a charitable or humanitarian pur-pose. Options include building houses or schools, working at an orphanage or refugee camp or partici-pating in an archeological dig, to name a few. It's not always "roughing it" either.

A company called Ambassadors for Children even offers a trip that includes a stay at a four-star hotel in Puerto Vallarta, Mexico, where three days of an eight-day trip are spent visiting an orphanage, library and preschool, giving participants a chance to combine purpose with pleasure.

Chapter 13
101 Aging Backwards Quick Tips

Easiest eating plan: Super-size your veggies and half-size everything else.

Coffee has more antioxidants than any food or drink in the average American diet, according to studies.

Order an appetizer as your entrée.

If you find yourself bingeing, don't just brush your teeth — floss and brush. All that hard work and the minty taste make you stop eating.

Freeze green tea or pomegranate juice and use them as ice cubes for the antioxidants.

Frozen grapes, bananas and strawberries taste like candy.

Be aware of the hidden calories in liquids like soda, juice and flavored water; read the label.

Organic fruits and vegetables have 40 percent more antioxidants than conventionally grown produce.

Frequent small meals keep you satisfied and help prevent bingeing.

Recognize the difference between hunger and thirst.

Use lemon juice to thin salad dressing — you'll use less and you won't lose any flavor.

Adding milk to a cup of tea can destroy its ability to protect against heart disease, according to research.

Concrete evidence from numerous studies reveals that smoking ages you by shortening the telomeres, or ends, of chromosomes.

Smokers who quit before age 50 cut their risk of dying in the next 15 years in half, according to the National Conference of State Legislatures.

Trick yourself into working out by dancing or jumping rope with your kids.

Do 100 Kegel exercises every day.

Weight training is essential after age 40.

Three travel essentials: jump rope, jog bra and sneakers.

Wear a pedometer; it makes you want to walk more.

When driving, hold your stomach in at the red lights, release at the green and remember to breathe.

Coconut oil is one of nature's best-kept secrets.

Take an Epsom salt bath to detoxify then rub coconut oil on before you towel off to give your skin a healthy glow and feel.

Small nips and tucks over time are better than one big overhaul when it comes to cosmetic surgery.

Accessorizing can go a long way toward updating your wardrobe.

Try facial exercises.

Choose a cosmetic surgeon who is an artist on the side – and a good one.

Laser hair removal really works for most people.

Over-washing your hair can strip it of essential oils.

Keep up with fashion, not fads.

Wearing fitted clothes can make you look slimmer, no matter what your size or shape.

You don't have to spend a fortune on clothes to look young — most young people can't afford high-priced, designer fashions.

Go to a department store when they have a bra-fitting event. Eighty-five percent of women wear the wrong bra size and/or style.

Trim nose hairs and excess "aging" hairs.

For precision results, use a magnifying mirror when applying eye makeup.

Wear a soft sleep bra at night. Don't let gravity do its thing.

According to experts, lip colors that have more blue in them make teeth look whiter.

Light lip color with gloss looks youthful.

Use hypoallergenic pillow liners to keep out bedbugs.

Use ultra soft pillowcases, and wash them frequently.

Sleep on your back or side, not your stomach.

Shorter nails look young.

French manicures look fresh and clean.

Keep up with your pedicures; even feet can show your age.

Keep grey roots invisible.

Keep your hair healthy, shiny and well cut.

Rinsing your hair in cold water closes the hair shaft, imparting youthful shine.

Catch rainwater from a summer shower in a bucket and use it to rinse your hair after shampooing. It feels great and softens hair.

Wearing a wig is a fast and fun way to change your look for the evening or anytime you want.

Remember to exfoliate to reveal younger skin.

Use SPF 35-50 every day on face, neck, chest and hands.

Self-tanners and bronzers can make you look thinner in minutes.

Makeup artists recommend wearing less makeup as we get older, not more.

Unscented baby wipes make great makeup removers in a rainstorm. I keep them in my car.

Highlight your best features.

Over-washing your face can strip skin of essential oils, exacerbating the natural dryness of aging skin.

Exfoliate lips by gently brushing them with a soft toothbrush, minus the toothpaste, of course.

Replace your toothbrush every three to four months or sooner if the bristles are frayed.

Gum disease can lead to heart attack and stroke.

For a quick pick-me-up, keep lightly scented cologne in the fridge and spritz to refresh.

Keep a little spray bottle of water in your purse to cool yourself when you're feeling hot or flushed.

From a flight attendant: put Neosporin around your nostrils before getting on a plane to kill any germs you might breathe in.

Keeping your nasal passages irrigated with saline solution has been shown to be effective in treating and preventing allergy symptoms and sinus infections.

A six-minute nap is all you need to rejuvenate and improve memory.

Getting your beauty rest can keep your weight down.

Melatonin is a natural supplement that can help you fall asleep faster and stay asleep.

Ten to 15 minutes of midday sun daily helps keep your vitamin D levels optimal.

Keep a wide-brimmed hat in your car — sun on your face ages you.

For an instant "escape," use earplugs to block out your surroundings, but not while driving.

Remember this saying: "90 percent of everything I worry about never happens."

When you feel overwhelmed, inhale for a count of four, hold for five and exhale for seven.

Talk to strangers, you might learn something. Dale Carnegie said it best: "Friendly people are lucky people."

Other people deserve their space, common courtesy and my respect.

Kneading dough is an excellent way to relieve stress.

Cleaning your house and your closet can be therapeutic.

Write down your goals, wants and needs.

Being as honest and authentic as possible keeps your stress level down.

To memorize phone numbers, sing them to the tune of a familiar song.

A one-day getaway, even in your own city, can rejuvenate.

Keeping up on current events helps you live in the present.

Talk less, listen more.

Holding onto anger ages you.

Hypnosis actually works for many people trying to break bad habits.

Join a club or organization.

Unclutter your life.

Write down the cute, funny things your kids say.

Sometimes escaping reality can be healthy; read books, see films, go to plays, etc.

Don't compare yourself to others.

Set small goals for yourself all day — it's very gratifying to achieve them.

Being productive can give you a great sense of accomplishment.

People who volunteer are the healthiest and live the longest, according to research.

Sponsoring a needy child is gratifying.

Treat yourself to fresh flowers — don't wait for someone else to send them.

Pets bring joy and energy into a house.

Meditate to reduce stress.

Visualize yourself looking and feeling younger.

Don't point out your flaws to anyone, even yourself.

There is almost nothing more stressful than being severely in debt.

Recognize the riches in your life that are not material.

Research has shown that practicing yoga can alleviate chronic pain.

Deep breathing spreads oxygen throughout the body, energizing every cell.

Keep your promises.

Chapter 14
Aging Backwards Favorites: Jackie's Fancy

Since I am the "Anti-Aging Petri Dish," I've tried lots and lots of anti-aging and beauty products, services and procedures over the years. I've compiled a list of some of my favorite things. I actually do use each and every one of these. Of course, I couldn't include every single "favorite" thing because that would take up a whole book by itself. Maybe that's the next Aging Backwards book?

Eyes:
ColorOn Instant Cream Eye Shadow – brilliant and beautiful.
Available: Sephora stores and coloronpro.com

Jane Iredale PurePressed Eye Shadows - pure minerals, gorgeous colors.
Available: Salons, spas, doctors' offices

Mac False Eyelashes - fluffy and natural, tons to pick from.
Available: Mac Cosmetics stores, counters and maccosmetics.com

SPINLASH – one of the greatest inventions of the 21st century, in my opinion. It's mascara with a spinning brush for perfect application. Sheer genius!
Available: spinlash.com

Maybelline Lash Stiletto™ Ultimate Length Washable Mascara - make my lashes long and gorgeous.
Available: Most retail stores and maybelline.com

Ardell Duo Eyelash Adhesive - it really sticks.
Available: Most beauty supply stores, see ardelllashes.com

Magnifying makeup mirror - for precision eye makeup application.
Available: Most retail stores

Garnier Nutritioniste Skin Renew Anti Sun Damage Eye Cream SPF 15 - the first eye cream at mass with SPF.
Available: Most retail stores and garnierusa.com

Osmotics Blue Copper 5 Firming Eye Repair - fixes crow's feet.
Available: Department stores and osmotics.com

Olay Definity Eye Illuminator - brightens eyes.
Available: Most pharmacy and retail stores, and olay.com

Colorescience Eye Candy Trio - great for concealing flaws.
Available: Spas, doctors' offices and find location at colorescience.com

Face:
Shel-Gel - My secret find with exotic ingredients from South America, plus vitamin E and collagen, for

beautiful Aging Backwards skin.
Available: shelgel.com

Per-fekt Skin Perfection Gel - as primer or foundation, skin looks airbrushed perfect.
Available: Sephora stores and perfektbeauty.com

DHC Deep Cleansing Oil - olive oil based, really cleans.
Available: dhccare.com

Solavie skin and haircare - it's the first unisex skin and hair line designed around the body's response to environmental conditions. No more worrying about skin type. Being a big-city girl, I use Urban.
Available: solavie.com

Facial Magic from Cynthia Rowland - facial exercise system that really works to lift and firm the face - these simple exercises really make me look younger!
Available: cynthiarowland.com

Mac Blot Film - blot that oily face, don't gunk it up with powder.
Available: Mac Cosmetics stores, counters and maccosmetics.com

Osmotics Age Prevention Protection Extreme SPF 40 - protects from sun damage, no residue.
Available: Department stores and osmotics.com

Olay Regenerist Micro-Sculpting Cream - chosen number one by Good Housekeeping Magazine.
Available: Most pharmacy and retail stores, and olay. com

Olay Professional Pro-X line - it works by resignaling your skin to repair the moisture barrier and boost the surface-cell turnover rate. I just know I love it!
Available: Check olay.com for locations

Cargo Cosmetics Blu-Ray High Definition Makeup – professional beauty, even if you're not on TV. The whole line is FAB, but my favorites are the concealer (the BEST!), the Mattifier and the mascara.
Available: cargocosmetics.com

Nars The Multiple - recommended by makeup expert Bruce Grayson, I like it for blush.
Available: Nars counters and narscosmetics.com

Lips:
Murad Soothing Skin and Lip Care - can't live without it for hydrated lips.
Available: Retail stores and murad.com

Cynthia Rowland Luscious Lips Lip Pump - plump, gorgeous lips the natural way.
Available: cynthiarowland.com

Mac Cosmetics Viva Glam Line of Lip Glass - every cent goes to Mac AIDS fund. Viva Glam V is my color.
Available: Mac Cosmetics stores, counters and mac-cosmetics.com

Revlon ColorStay Lipliner - lasts long and great price.
Available: Most pharmacy, retail and grocery stores,
see revlon.com

Hair:
PureOlogy NanoWorks Shampoo & Conditioner -
super expensive, but gorgeous results.
Available: Salons and some beauty supply stores

L'Oreal Excellence Creme Haircolor - okay, it has
chemicals, but it covers my gray.
Available: Wherever L'Oreal hair color is sold, see loreal.
com

Moroccanoil - smoothes, adds shine, truly amazing product.
Available: Salons, see moroccanoil.com

Pantene Relaxed & Natural Breakage Defense Deep
Conditioning Mask - hair feels great.
Available: Wherever Pantene products are sold, see
pantene.com

Body:
Ageless Perfume - the world's first anti-aging perfume
that incorporates the essence of pink grapefruit with
pomegranate, mango, jasmine and musk - a combination that studies prove makes men perceive women as
eight years younger.
Available: agelessperfume.com

Bethesda Sunscreen Soap - SPF sun protection in a
soap bar with vitamins. Why didn't I think of this?
Available: bethesdaskincare.com

CherryPharm All Natural Juice – 50 cherries in each bottle for antioxidants – even helps improve sleep.
Available: cherrypharm.com

Vital Choice Wild Seafood and Organics - the freshest, most delectable fish you ever tasted, straight from Alaska. I know the founder, Randy Hartnell, personally.
Available: vitalchoice.com

Lush Karma Soap - handmade and smells divine.
Available: Lush stores and lush.com

Yes to Carrots Shower Gel - organic ingredients combined with charity: provides seeds to farms.
Available: Walgreens, Duane Reade, Ulta Beauty and Home Shopping Network (HSN)

Supplements:
Skin Defense Complex by Astavita - Beauty from within! Don't HIDE the signs of aging - DEFY them. I love this product! Two tiny, easy-to-swallow softgels daily and I'm Aging Backwards from the inside, out!
Available: http://www.astavita.com/topical.html

LifeVantage's Protandim - Aging Backwards at the cellular level with Superoxide Dismutase- the fountain of youth?
Available: protandim.com

Corvalen Bioenergy Ribose – good for lots of things, see the supplements chapter. I love the chocolate taste of the chewable.
Available: bioenergy.com

Astavita Professional AstaREAL Astaxanthin – guards against the effects of excessive free radicals.
Available: astavita.com

Omega-Cure Extra Virgin Fish Oil - no fishy taste or smell, there's nothing else like it.
Available: omega-cure.com

Real Advantage Ultimate Bionic Plus - makes my workouts worth the effort.
Available: realadvantagenutrients.com

Dr. Ron Wheeler's Bladder Balance - no more running to the bathroom.
Available: peenuts.com

Dr. Sears' Primal Force Accel CoQ10 - keeps my brain sharp.
Available: primalforce.net/catalog

Mellow Tone with Melatonin - Like a breath strip -I sleep like a baby.
Available: Ask your doctor, see mellow-tone.com

Fitness:
Dr. Al Sears' PACE program - shortest workout with best results.
Available: alsearsmd.com

The Firm - these women are fabulous. I want to look like them when I grow up.
Available: Retail stores and firmdirect.com

Teeter Hang Ups Inversion Table - hanging upside down decompresses and relaxes me.
Available: Some retail stores and teeterhangups.com

JumpSnap Ropeless Jump Rope - the ultimate in portable workouts (besides your feet) and no rope to trip on. I like that it comes with weights you can add to the handles.
Available: jumpsnap.com

Miscellaneous:
Merl Reagle's Sunday Crosswords - Okay, so Merl's my friend, but he does make the best puzzles on earth.
Available: sundaycrosswords.com

Skinny Songs - Fun, catchy songs that make me want to go on a diet, even though I don't need one.
Available: skinnysongs.com

Solerra Sunless Tanning Mitt - I love this self-tanner mitt because I don't have to get the product on my hands and I get a beautiful bronze glow.
Available: solerra.com

Closet Fetish Shoe Boxes - they're pretty and they keep me organized - that's not easy.
Available: closetfetish.com

SmartLipo - I got rid of fat with a laser that also tightens skin.
Available: Ask your doctor, see smartlipo.com

VelaShape - I got rid of cellulite and shrank my waist without surgery.
Available: Ask your doctor, see velashape.com

Triniti by Syneron - I got rid of sun spots, got my skin tightened and collagen stimulated all at the same time without pain.
Available: Ask your doctor, see syneron.com

Emotional Freedom Techniques (EFT, see Chapter 10) – I like EFT for coping with stress, worry and pain.
Available: emofree.com - download a free guide
Also at: tryitoneverything.com

Fezelry Jewelry - gorgeous, affordable designs to help you accessorize your wardrobe.
Available: fezelryjewelry.com

Aging Backwards Crossword Puzzle
By Merl Reagle
Answers

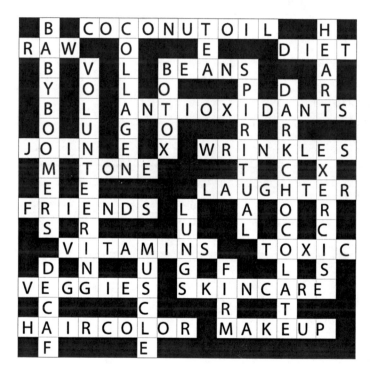

Expert Opinion Bios

The people I've quoted throughout the book for their expert opinion are among the top experts in their respective fields, including anti-aging, medical, beauty, fashion, cosmeceutical, nutraceutical, fitness, health and dental. I personally interviewed them for this book and I am honored to share their expertise with you.

Dana Cuculici, DMD

Dr. Dana Cuculici has been practicing dentistry for almost 20 years. Her practice includes a wide range of dental procedures, including comprehensive dentistry, implant restorations, crowns, bridges as well as other cosmetic and restorative procedures. Dr. Dana utilizes the latest technology available in dentistry today. These modalities include digital x-rays, intra-oral cameras, cosmetic video imaging and multimedia patient education. Dr. Dana has lived in Transylvania, Casablanca, Morocco and California. She is fluent in German, Romanian, French and English. All these experiences help her to understand and communicate with people from different backgrounds. She was educated in Romania and at U. C. L. A. in California.

Bruce Fife, C.N., N.D.
Dr. Bruce Fife, C.N., N.D., is an author, speaker, certified nutritionist, and naturopath. He has written 23 books including Coconut Cures, The Coconut Oil Miracle, and Eat Fat, Look Thin. He is the publisher and editor of the Healthy Ways Newsletter. He serves as the president of the Coconut Research Center (www. coconutresearchcenter.org), a non-profit organization which is dedicated to educating the public about the health and nutritional aspects of coconut.

Joel Fuhrman, M.D.
Joel Fuhrman, M.D., is a board-certified family physician, best-selling author, and one of the country's leading experts on nutritional medicine. He speaks to audiences at conferences, seminars, and corporate events throughout the United States and Canada. He addresses other physicians at hospital grand rounds and has lectured at benefits for the American Heart Association and the U.S. Olympic Team. Dr. Fuhrman has appeared in hundreds of magazines, on the radio, and on television including: Good Morning America (ABC), The Today Show (NBC), Good Day New York (FOX), The Food Network, CNN, UPN, and the Discovery Channel. His books include: Eat To Live, Cholesterol Protection for Life, and Disease Proof Your Child. His newest book, Eat For Health, was published in April 2008. Dr. Fuhrman teaches nutrition excellence is not only preventative, but is also the most effective therapeutic interventions for most chronic medical conditions. At DrFuhrman.com he supplies health and nutrition information and answers people's health and nutrition questions.

Bruce Grayson
Bruce Grayson is one of the few makeup artists who
was born and raised in Los Angeles. Exposed to
makeup at an early age by his father, Dave Grayson,
he realized he could apply his love of art and painting
to faces. He quickly became one of the most request-
ed makeup artists in print and television. Hollywood
producers were quick to hire Bruce for his talent at
making celebrities look and feel beautiful. He has an
incredible understanding of lighting and how to adjust
makeup so that his clients look their best in film, television and print. From his work as department head
on television shows such as The Academy Awards and
The Emmys, to the sitcom Just Shoot Me and his work
on magazines such as Vanity Fair, he is constantly hired
for his level of professionalism. His passion and enthusiasm for the art of beauty makeup is contagious.

David A. Kekich
Mr. Kekich founded the country's largest life insurance
master general agency, which raised $3.1 billion of
premium income for First Executive Corp., co-founded a major financial services company and arranged
venture capital funding for private companies for 11
years. He is a recognized expert on private investing
and authored the venture capital handbook "How The
Rich Get Richer With Quiet Private Investments." Mr.
Kekich founded both public and private companies,
was engaged as a consultant and served as director
to numerous private and public corporations. He also
sold and developed real estate. In 1999, Mr. Kekich
founded the "Maximum Life Foundation," a 501(c)(3)
corporation dedicated to reversing human aging and

aging related diseases. In 2006, he co-founded Stem Cell Products, LLC. Mr. Kekich also authored "Life Extension Express," a how-to book for extreme life extension. He serves as a Board Member of the American Aging Association.

Ronald M. Klatz, M.D., D.O.

Dr. Ronald Klatz is recognized as a leading authority in the new clinical science of anti-aging medicine. He is the physician founder and President of the American Academy of Anti-Aging Medicine Inc. ("A4M"), a non-profit medical organization dedicated to the advancement of technology to detect, prevent, and treat aging related disease and to promote research into methods to retard and optimize the human aging process. Dr. Klatz has authored numerous books, including the nonfiction bestseller Grow Young with HGH (HarperCollins), Stopping the Clock: Longevity for the New Millennium, Ten Weeks to a Younger You, New Anti-Aging Secrets for Maximum Lifespan, Brain Fitness (Doubleday), Hormones of Youth, Seven Anti-Aging Secrets, Advances in Anti-Aging, Stopping the Clock, and more. Dr. Klatz is a graduate of Florida Technological University. Dr. Klatz received the Doctor of Medicine (M.D.) Degree from the Central America Health Sciences University, School of Medicine. He received his Doctor of Osteopathic Medicine and Surgery (D.O.) degree from the College of Osteopathic Medicine and Surgery (Des Moines, Iowa). A consultant to the biotechnology industry and a respected advisor to several members of the U.S. Congress and others on Capitol Hill, Dr. Klatz devotes much of his time to research and to the development of advanced

biosciences for the benefit of humanity. Go to www.
worldhealth.net for more information.

Lauren Messiah
As the Fashion and Beauty Manager, Lauren Messiah is
the ThisNext's fashion trendsetter. She keeps her finger on the pulse of what's hot by interacting daily with
more than one million monthly visitors to the ThisNext
community. Lauren uses her fashionista insights to
drive strategic content development for ThisNext and
dish out fashion/beauty advice on her blog at www.
AskFashionKitty.com. She has been a part of the style
world for nearly ten years (if you want to get technical
– since birth) and resides in Los Angeles with her 75
pairs of jeans—and no, there is no such thing as too
much denim. When she isn't pinpointing what the next
great fashion/beauty item will be, she can be found
on the yoga mat, at the gym or feeding her obsession
with cats.

Roger Y. Murray, M.D.
Dr. Roger Murray, M.D. is an Orlando, Florida-based
cosmetic surgeon, specializing in minimally invasive
cosmetic surgery and is an expert in scar minimization
techniques, aesthetics and anti-aging. He has been in
medical practice for 25 years and has recently trademarked Telemorx™, a daily supplement he created to
help provide a boost of energy for patients who com-
plained of feeling tired and run down. He graduated
from Medical University of South Carolina, after which
he did an internship in Internal Medicine and residency
in Family Practice. He became board certified in Family Practice and recently took his boards in Phlebology.

He has been the past Vice President of the American Society of Phlebectomy and recently served his term as President of the American College of Phlebology Surgery Section. He co-authored the book Practice without Fear, wrote the book Forever Young and Healthy and is working on another book entitled Tele-Kinesthesiology. He currently teaches cosmetic procedures in his office and teaches physicians how to enhance the face with Sculptra (Sanofi-Aventis).

Sangeeta Pati, M.D., FACOG
Dr. Pati is a Georgetown University trained physician who practiced traditional and holistic medicine for fifteen years in the Washington D.C. area. She has practiced extensively in the U.S. and internationally including serving as Medical director for a 350-employee non-profit organization. Dr. Pati is multi-lingual and is renowned in her field, having authored numerous scientific articles and addressing audiences both nationally and internationally. She is recognized by physicians internationally as a foremost authority in the field of Bio-Identical Hormone Replacement Therapy. Dr. Pati holds board certifications from the American Board of Ob/Gyn and American Anti-Aging Board of Medicine.

Francine Porter
Francine Porter is the Founder, CEO, and Creative Director of Osmotics, a prestige cosmetic line specializing in anti-aging cosmeceutical skin care. She is also responsible for product development and is the spokesperson and corporate image figure for the company. Francine, an Atlanta native, has endured skin sensitivity from the age of 14. As a result, she

has made a personal commitment to developing the purest and most effective skin care products available. Through extensive study and research, she has achieved a famed position in the cosmetic arena. Following Francine's innovative vision, Osmotics has introduced some of the most revolutionary new concepts in the field of anti-aging skincare. Francine is recognized as an expert in the area of cosmetics and skin care, and is sought around the world for her training, knowledge and expertise.

Merl Reagle

Merl Reagle made his first crossword at age 6 and sold his first crossword to The New York Times when he was only 16. Games Magazine has called him "the best Sunday crossword puzzle creator in America" and his popular syndicated crossword, which has been described as having a "Far Side" sense of humor, appears every Sunday in the Washington Post, Los Angeles Times, San Francisco Chronicle, Philadelphia Inquirer, and many other major newspapers. He is featured prominently in the hit documentary Wordplay (along with President Bill Clinton, comedy host Jon Stewart, and others). The documentary was the third most critically acclaimed film of 2006. He has appeared on Nightline with Ted Koppel, The Oprah Show and even an episode of The Simpsons, which revolves around Lisa entering a crossword contest in Springfield. Merl also made all the crosswords seen in the episode. He is the author of 12 critically acclaimed volumes of Sunday crossword puzzles and he syndicates an "eraser-free" sudoku to newspapers around the country. Merl lives in Tampa, Florida, with his better half,

Marie Haley, whom he describes as "the real brains of the outfit." He's been playing keyboards since he was 10 years old, collects movie soundtracks, and writes music in a style he calls "detective rock."

Ray Sahelian, M.D.

Ray Sahelian, M.D., obtained a Bachelors of Science degree in nutrition from Drexel University and completed his doctoral training at Thomas Jefferson Medical School, both in Philadelphia. He is certified by the American Board of Family Medicine. A popular and respected physician and medical writer, Dr. Sahelian is internationally recognized as a moderate voice in the evaluation of natural supplements. What makes Dr. Sahelian different than almost all other doctors who write about supplements is that he actually tests on himself various herbs and nutrients in varying dosages to determine what kind of effect they have. It is this experimental and experiential method that has provided him with significant insights into herbs and supplements that few other medical doctors have discovered. Dr. Sahelian has been seen on television programs including NBC Today, NBC Nightly News, CBS This Morning, Dateline NBC, and CNN, quoted by countless major magazines such as Newsweek, Modern Maturity, Health, and newspapers including USA Today, Los Angeles Times, Washington Post, and Le Monde (France). Millions of radio listeners nationwide hear him discuss the latest research on health. He is in private practice in Los Angeles, CA.

Al Sears, M.D.

Al Sears, MD sees patients at his integrative clinic and research center in Florida where he has developed novel exercise and nutritional systems transforming the lives of over 20,000 patients. With over 500 articles and six books in the fields of alternative medicine, anti-aging and nutritional supplementation, Dr. Sears enjoys a worldwide readership and has appeared on over 50 national radio programs, ABC News, CNN and ESPN. He is the author of PACE: Rediscover Your Native Fitness and The Doctor's Heart Cure. Dr. Sears is a board certified clinical nutrition specialist and was appointed to the international panel of experts at Health Sciences Institute, (HSI) a worldwide information service for alternative nutritional therapies. Dr. Sears is a member of the American Academy of Anti-Aging Medicine and is Board Certified in Anti-Aging Medicine. He is a member of the American College of Sports Medicine and the National Youth Sports Coaches Association.

Stephen T. Sinatra, M.D.

Stephen T. Sinatra, M.D., F.A.C.C., F.A.C.N., C.N.S., C.B.T., is a board-certified cardiologist, certified bio-energetic psychotherapist, and certified as a nutrition and anti-aging specialist. He integrates psychological, nutraceutical and electroceutical therapies in the matrix of healing. He is a fellow in the American College of Cardiology and the American College of Nutrition. He writes a national monthly newsletter entitled Heart, Health and Nutrition and his latest book, Metabolic Cardiology/The Sinatra Solution was recently released.

Jacqueline Tarrant
After more than 20 years of experience in hair care, Jacqueline Tarrant founded the Chicago-based Style Infinity Hair Trauma Center (HTC). Style Infinity HTC employs a comprehensive approach to aid hair regeneration, which includes a clinically proven nutritional supplement, FDA proven topical component and technologically advanced Low Laser Light Therapy (LLLT), which utilizes Light Emitting Diode (LED) lasers to deliver light emanating energy directly from each bulb. As the former product development specialist and Director of Education for L'Oreal USA, Jacqueline is known as an innovative leader and team builder with a tremendous enthusiasm for the beauty and hair care industry. During her career, she has also successfully owned and operated full-service beauty salons in Baltimore since 1985. Her salon has provided her with years of hands-on experience, which she is able to employ in her assessment and treatment of Style Infinity HTC clientele. During her tenure at L'Oreal, Jacqueline served as key spokeswoman, making numerous style & beauty appearances nationwide on ABC, NBC, CBS and the Fox Network. Her media credits also include such print publications as Seventeen, Cosmopolitan, Essence & the Wall Street Journal.

Roger Teeter
Roger and Jennifer Teeter founded Hang Ups Inversion Products in 1981 and have been dedicated to manufacturing quality inversion products ever since. Inversion has changed Roger's life; he is dedicated to sharing his knowledge of inversion and quality products with the world. Roger and Jenny first "dis-

covered" inversion at a water ski tournament in 1980. At the time, Roger was suffering from severe back problems resulting from his job as a professional water skier and from an auto accident. In constant pain, he continued to compete professionally, forced to wear a large back brace with metal rods. He had tried many forms of therapy to help manage his pain and discovered that by inverting (hanging upside down), he was able to relieve his back pain and begin on the road to recovery. Roger began inverting in 1980 and has been doing it ever since. He credits inversion for keeping him pain free, healthy and active. Roger saw a need for safe, quality equipment and decided to start a company dedicated to manufacturing inversion products. Sky's the Limit (STL) entered the inversion market in 1981 with the Hang Ups inversion products. Teeter Hang Ups is the only company in the world to manufacture inversion products continuously since 1981.

Lyda D. Tymiak, M.D., P.A.

In 1980, Dr Tymiak founded Gulfcoast Eye Care in Palm Harbor, Florida, a general ophthalmology practice treating all eye disorders both medical and surgical and specializing in refractive cataract and implant surgery, as well as facial plastic surgery. In 2004, Timeless MD Spa was added, offering state of the art facial rejuvenation using lasers and light based treatment and Elos technology, fillers and Botox. Body shaping with Velashape was added in 2008. Dr Tymiak received her BA degree from Boston University and an MD degree from Albert Einstein College of Medicine. She completed an internship in Internal Medicine and a residency in ophthalmology at University of South Florida, followed by

Board Certification in Ophthalmology. Dr Tymiak is an affiliate of Cenegenics Age Reversal Medicine Institute. Herteaching appointments include Associate Professor of Ophthalmology at the University of South Florida, National Education Faculty for Allergan, and faculty for Syneron teaching workshops. She has appeared on numerous TV shows, news broadcasts including Daytime TV featuring Elos technology. Her professional memberships include American Academy of Ophthalmology, Florida Society of Ophthalmology, Pinellas County Medical Society, where she has served on the Board of Governors, American Medical Women's Association, American Medical Association, Ukranian Medical Association. Dr Tymiak was past President of the Tampa Bay Ophthalmological Society. Her daughter, Dr Andrea Cottrell, joined the practice in June 2007 forming the first mother/daughter EYE MD team.

Acknowledgments

Many people have supported me during the writing of this book, both personally and professionally. Thanks to my son, Trent, for his loving support and patience throughout this process.

Additional thanks:
To my family, Dr. Deborah Willig, Dr. Susan Fan, David Willig, Esquire, Ray Willig, Steven Camelo, Devon Fan and Colby Fan. An extra special thank you to my brother, David Willig, for his exceptional legal acumen and business advice.

To all of the experts who generously gave their time and insights for the Expert Opinion quotes.

To Merl Reagle for his original Aging Backwards Crossword Puzzle.

To Xavier Rivera for designing the covers and inside layout of the book and to Pamela Huff for editing.

To Linda LaMonte, Brenda Cutler Boone, Dr. Kathy Clements, Kendall Almerico, Tamra Nashman, Joe Monko, Dr. Richard Silver, Kevin and Kaysie O'Donnell, Patti Tilchin, Patrick Mixon, Dawn Marie Campbell, Dr. Bart Rademaker, Rose Marie Lawand, Brian Greenberg, Wesley Hein, Gregory Yorke, Billy Montana,

Sandi McKenna, Kumar Ramani, Mo and Lance Eppley, Melanie Segala, Christian Schwier, Tony Wagner, Susan Larkin, Paul and Tamara Meek, Pam Dover, Scott Siskin and others too numerous to mention.

About the Author

Jackie Silver is Aging Backwards and she shares her secrets, tips and shortcuts for looking and feeling young on her Web site, AgingBackwards.com, in her book, on TV, on radio, in print, online and in person. She's the Aging Backwards expert on the syndicated television show, Daytime; the beauty editor for Clear Channel's Mix 100.7 Nancy & Chris Mornings in Tampa Bay; frequent guest on Familynet TV's Everyday With Marcus and Lisa; weekly columnist for The Tampa Tribune and a sought-after speaker.

She founded Aging Backwards, LLC, in 2006 to educate the public about the latest innovations in the anti-aging industry. She has more than 25 years of experience in broadcasting and she combines her natural reporter's curiosity with her desire to help people look and feel younger.

She is a member of the American Academy of Anti-Aging Medicine, the American Heart Association Community Board, Screen Actors Guild and the American Federation of Television and Radio Artists.
Feel free to contact the author at **jackie@agingbackwards.com** or visit the Web site, **agingbackwards.com**.

Free Offer! We'd like to offer a free ten-minute phone consultation with Jackie. To redeem your free consultation, send an email to: **jackie@agingbackwards.com** and put **FREE CONSULT** in the subject line.